Ear, Nose and Throat at a Glance

The new book is also available as an ebook.
For more details, please see www.wiley.com/buy/9781444330878
or scan this QR code:

Ear, Nose and Throat at a Glance

Nazia Munir

Consultant ENT Surgeon
University Hospital Aintree, Liverpool, UK

Ray Clarke

Consultant ENT Surgeon
Alder Hey Hospital, Liverpool, UK
Associate Postgraduate Dean, Mersey Deanery, UK

WILEY-BLACKWELL

A John Wiley & Sons, Ltd., Publication

This edition first published 2013, © Nazia Munir and Ray Clarke

Blackwell Publishing was acquired by John Wiley & Sons in February 2007. Blackwell's publishing program has been merged with Wiley's global Scientific, Technical and Medical business to form Wiley-Blackwell.

Registered office: John Wiley & Sons, Ltd, The Atrium, Southern Gate, Chichester, West Sussex, PO19 8SQ, UK

Editorial offices: 9600 Garsington Road, Oxford, OX4 2DQ, UK
The Atrium, Southern Gate, Chichester, West Sussex, PO19 8SQ, UK
111 River Street, Hoboken, NJ 07030-5774, USA

For details of our global editorial offices, for customer services and for information about how to apply for permission to reuse the copyright material in this book please see our website at www.wiley.com/wiley-blackwell.

Library of Congress Cataloging-in-Publication Data
Munir, Nazia.
  Ear, nose, and throat at a glance / Nazia Munir, Ray Clarke.
      p. ; cm.
  Includes bibliographical references and index.
  ISBN 978-1-4443-3087-8 (pbk. : alk. paper)
  I. Clarke, Ray (Raymond). II. Title.
  [DNLM: 1. Otorhinolaryngologic Diseases–Handbooks. 2. Ear–physiopathology–Handbooks.
3. Nose–physiopathology–Handbooks. 4. Pharynx–physiopathology–Handbooks. WV 39]
  617.5'23–dc23
                            2012032720

A catalogue record for this book is available from the British Library.

Wiley also publishes its books in a variety of electronic formats. Some content that appears in print may not be available in electronic books.

Cover image: ALAIN POL, ISM/SCIENCE PHOTO LIBRARY
Cover design by Nathan Harris

Set in 9.5/12 Times by Toppan Best-set Premedia Limited
Printed and bound in Malaysia by Vivar Printing Sdn Bhd

1   2013

Contents

Preface

'Teach these boys and girls nothing but Facts. Facts alone are wanted in life. Plant nothing else, and root out everything else.' Thus speaks the fearsome teacher Thomas Gradgrind in *Hard Times.* (1)

Unlike Dickens's Mr. Gradgrind, we are mindful that students have a finite capacity for facts and we have tried not to overburden them. This book is deliberately short. We present the essential tenets of a complex and diverse specialty in a simple, visual way with minimal discussion of contentious areas or rare conditions and with maximum focus on the core principles. The *At a Glance* format with its emphasis on visual learning and on the presentation of information in a concise easy to follow format with minimum extraneous text is ideally suited to ENT. Ours is a highly 'visual' specialty; multiple clinical signs are apparent on simple inspection using a light source and inexpensive equipment. The capacity to take a good history, listening carefully to what the patient says allied with a torch and a good otoscope will serve both student and GP well for nearly all of the conditions we describe and for most of her/his career. Ideally, we want students to use this book to supplement the knowledge and skills they gain during even a very short attachment to an ENT unit or to a general practice, where many of the conditions we describe will be readily seen.

Long experience of teaching medical students and listening to their feedback have left us in no doubt that even the most enthusiastic and organised undergraduate struggles with the sheer volume of information bombarding her/him as the final medical examination approaches. Clinical practice is now so diverse and so specialised that multiple subspecialties and experts rightly want to impart some of the basics of their sphere of practice to their young charges. We are cognisant that many students have virtually dispensed with text books as there are good quality teaching resources online and in various electronic formats. This barrage of competing sources of information can be bewildering; it is easy to get demoralised and feel you are laden down with facts, hence the need for a concise summary that covers all of the ENT that might reasonably be expected of a newly qualified doctor.

We have included some basic applied anatomy and physiology alongside the clinical material; experience has also taught us that few undergraduates now have the confident grasp of detailed anatomy and physiology that was the norm a generation ago. There is just too much to learn and we have focused only on those aspects of basic science of immediate clinical relevance.

We include a brief self assessment section not because we want students to commit the text to memory but because many students tell us they find this an invaluable learning aid.

ENT covers a huge breadth of pathology and is nowadays composed of several subspecialties. We have tried to distill it down to the basics. We hope this little book communicates some of our enthusiasm for a fabulous specialty and that the student is stimulated not only to learn but to enjoy his/her all-too-short time on the ENT unit.

Nazia Munir
Ray Clarke

1. *Hard Times, Charles Dickens 1854.*

Acknowledgements

Some of the clinical photographs were kindly supplied by Mr Sankalap Tandon, Consultant Head and Neck Surgeon, University Hospital Aintree, Liverpool, and Mr Peter Bull, Emeritus Consultant ENT Surgeon, Sheffield.

1 Applied anatomy of the ear

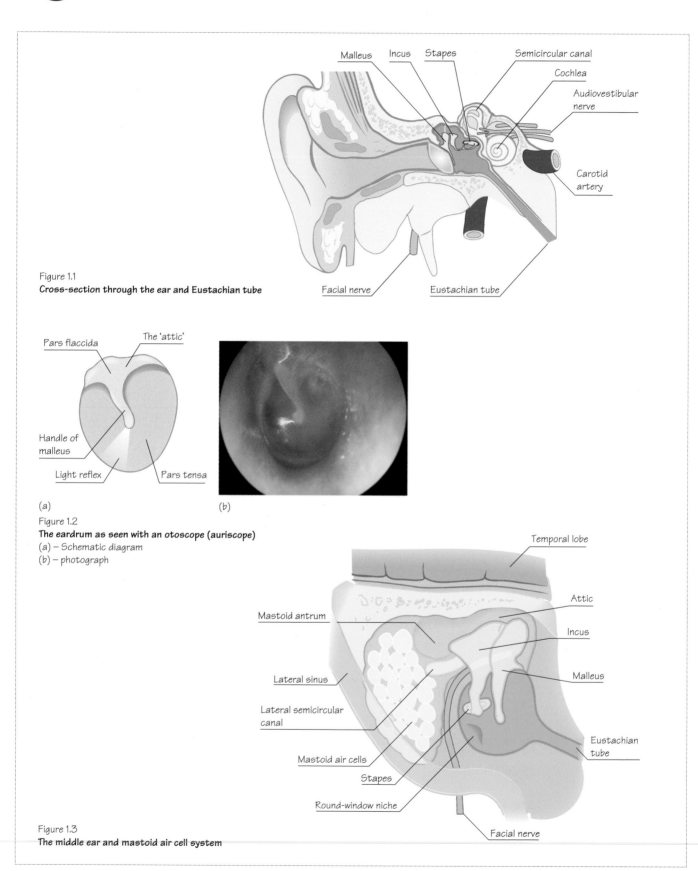

Figure 1.1
Cross-section through the ear and Eustachian tube

Malleus   Incus   Stapes   Semicircular canal   Cochlea   Audiovestibular nerve   Carotid artery   Facial nerve   Eustachian tube

Figure 1.2
The eardrum as seen with an otoscope (auriscope)
(a) – Schematic diagram
(b) – photograph

Pars flaccida   The 'attic'   Handle of malleus   Light reflex   Pars tensa

(a)   (b)

Figure 1.3
The middle ear and mastoid air cell system

Temporal lobe   Attic   Incus   Malleus   Eustachian tube   Facial nerve   Round-window niche   Stapes   Mastoid air cells   Lateral semicircular canal   Lateral sinus   Mastoid antrum

Ear, Nose and Throat at a Glance, First Edition. Nazia Munir and Ray Clarke.

The ear

The ear has three divisions:
1 The outer (external) ear
2 The middle ear
3 The inner ear

External ear

The external ear is made up of (Figure 1.1):
• The pinna
• The external auditory meatus (ear canal)
• Lateral portion of tympanic membrane (ear drum)

The outer (lateral) part of the external ear has a cartilaginous skeleton and the deep (medial) part has a bony skeleton: both are lined by skin. Skin overlying the lateral portion contains hair follicles and sebaceous and wax glands, which are all absent in the medial portion.

The tympanic membrane forms a boundary between the external and middle ears and is divided into the stiffer pars tensa below and the less rigid pars flaccida above (Figure 1.2).

Middle ear

The middle ear is an air-filled space behind the tympanic membrane that contains the ossicles (bones of hearing): malleus, incus and stapes (Figures 1.1 and 1.3). The ossicles form the ossicular chain, which amplifies and transmits sound vibrations to the inner ear.

The Eustachian tube forms a link between the middle ear and nasopharynx. The facial nerve (cranial nerve VII) also runs through the middle ear. Posteriorly, the mastoid air cell system also opens directly into the middle ear (Figures 1.1 and 1.3).

Inner ear

The inner ear comprises (Figure 1.1):
• The part of the middle ear behind the pars flaccida is called the 'attic'.
• The cochlea – this part of the inner ear creates electrical impulses in the cochlear nerve (cranial nerve VIII). These impulses are relayed to the brain to be perceived as sound.
• The vestibule and labyrinth (semicircular canals) – these are involved in balance control.

Anatomical relations of the ear

The ear is close to some important structures which can be involved if infection or disease spread:
• *Eustachian tube* (Figures 1.1 and 1.3) This is a part bony and part cartilaginous tube lined with ciliated epithelium that connects the middle ear space with the **nasopharynx**. Infection in the nose and pharynx can easily track up this tube to the middle ear, which is really a part of the upper respiratory tract. The Eustachian tube is especially important in children – it is wider, shorter and more upright than in adults. Gently hold your nose, close your mouth and try to exhale – you will feel air entering your middle ear via the Eustachian tube.
• *Mastoid air cell system* The mastoid process is a bony lump behind the pinna that contains a honeycomb network of epithelium-lined air cells (mastoid air cells). The mastoid air cell system opens directly into the middle ear cleft (Figure 1.3). Infection can track in here to cause 'mastoiditis' (see Figure 8.3).
• *Middle cranial fossa* This contains the temporal lobe of the brain and sits just above the middle ear so meningitis and brain abscess are possible complications of ear infection.
• *Venous sinuses* These surround the brain and carry blood to the neck veins and are also closely related to the middle ear and mastoid. Infection can propagate and result in potentially fatal cavernous sinus thrombosis.
• *Facial nerve* The seventh cranial nerve runs through the mastoid and the middle ear. It supplies the muscles of facial expression and is at risk in ear infections and in some types of ear surgery.

TIPS FOR EAR EXAMINATION

• Look at the pinna and the mastoid and check for swellings, scars and colour change.
• Use a good quality otoscope (auriscope) to obtain a view of the eardrum. Use the biggest speculum that will comfortably fit and do not put it in too far.
• You may need to straighten the ear canal by pulling the pinna upwards and backwards to help fit the speculum in.
• Note the condition of the skin of the external ear and try to get a good look at the eardrum in a systematic manner.
• Complete examination includes tuning fork tests, hearing assessment, assessment of facial nerve function and post-nasal space examination to look at the Eustachian tube opening.

Clinical practice point

If you cannot obtain a good view of the eardrum using an otoscope, gently manipulate the pinna. Do not put the speculum in too far.

2 Physiology of hearing

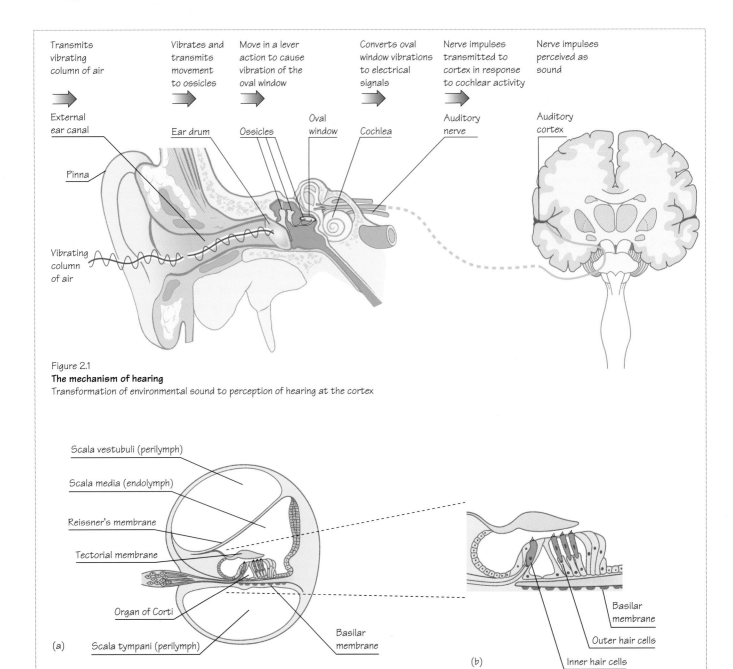

Transmits vibrating column of air ⇨

Vibrates and transmits movement to ossicles ⇨

Move in a lever action to cause vibration of the oval window ⇨

Converts oval window vibrations to electrical signals ⇨

Nerve impulses transmitted to cortex in response to cochlear activity ⇨

Nerve impulses perceived as sound

External ear canal

Ear drum

Ossicles

Oval window

Cochlea

Auditory nerve

Auditory cortex

Pinna

Vibrating column of air

Figure 2.1

The mechanism of hearing

Transformation of environmental sound to perception of hearing at the cortex

Scala vestubuli (perilymph)

Scala media (endolymph)

Reissner's membrane

Tectorial membrane

Organ of Corti

(a) Scala tympani (perilymph)

Basilar membrane

Basilar membrane

Outer hair cells

Inner hair cells

(b)

Figure 2.2

The fine structure of the cochlea showing hair cells and the auditory nerve

(a) Cross-section of the cochlea. The scala tympani and scala vestibuli are filled with perilymph, and the scala media is filled with endolymph. It is separated from the scala tympani by Reissner's membrane and from the scala vestibuli by the basilar membrane which supports the organ of Corti
(b) Diagram representing the organ of Corti. The entire length of the cochlea contains one row of inner hair cells and three rows of outer hair cells

The ear has two physiological functions: hearing and the maintenance of balance (see Chapter 12).

Physiology of hearing

'Hearing' is a vital part of our communication; speech, conversation, music, traffic and a host of other sounds are an integral part of our lives. Hearing is a complex physiological process starting with sound energy vibrating a column of air in the external ear and the bones that surround the ear. This in turn causes the eardrum and the attached ossicles to move in a delicate sequence and set up fluid movements in the cochlea or inner ear (Figure 2.1).

Highly specialised cells in the cochlea (hair cells) create electrical impulses that are then transmitted via the auditory nerve to the auditory cortex – the part of the brain concerned with receiving and interpreting sound (Figure 2.2).

This sequence can be interrupted at many levels, causing varying degrees of deafness.

Types of hearing loss

Conductive hearing loss

Interruption to the hearing mechanism in the external ear or the middle ear prevents 'conduction' of sound energy to the cochlea resulting in hearing loss (conductive hearing loss). If the cochlea is working well, vibrations from the environment will still get to the inner ear and the auditory nerve. Some hearing (often quite good hearing) is therefore still possible.

Sensorineural hearing loss

If the hearing process is interrupted at the cochlea or in the auditory nerve – for example, if the hair cells are damaged – then the hearing loss is referred to as 'sensorineural'. It can be complete (i.e. the patient is profoundly deaf), and is much more difficult to treat.

Clinical practice point

Always try to distinguish between conductive and sensorineural hearing loss. Tuning fork tests will help but definitive audiometric assessments such as pure tone audiometry are essential (see Chapter 3).

3 Testing the hearing

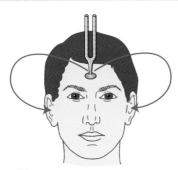

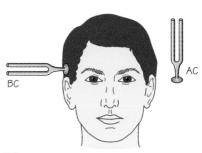

Figure 3.1
Weber test
Place the base of a vibrating tuning fork in the middle of the patient's forehead. Ask her/him where she/he hears the sound better – on the right, on the left, or in the middle. In the middle is 'Weber central', to the right is 'Weber right' and to the left is 'Weber left'. In a left conductive deafness the Weber is left. In a left sensorineural deafness it is right. This is not completely reliable but can be very helpful

Figure 3.2
Rinne test
This compares air conduction (AC) with bone conduction (BC). Place the vibrating tuning fork adjacent to the patient's ear canal (AC). Now place the base on the mastoid tip (BC) and ask her/him which sound is louder. If AC is louder than BC this is recorded as 'Rinne positive'. If BC is louder, this is 'Rinne negative'. Rinne negative usually means a conductive loss. Normal hearing results in Rinne positive (i.e AC>BC), and Rinne is also positive in sensorineural hearing loss

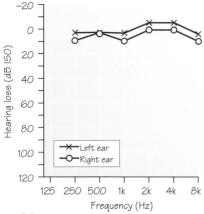

Figure 3.3a
Pure tone audiogram – normal

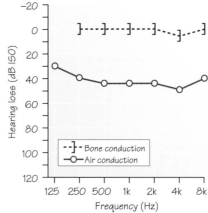

Figure 3.3b
Pure tone audiogram (right ear) – shows the pattern of a conductive hearing loss. Note that air conduction is much worse than bone conduction. The difference is termed the 'air bone gap'

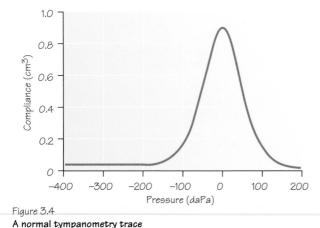

Figure 3.4
A normal tympanometry trace

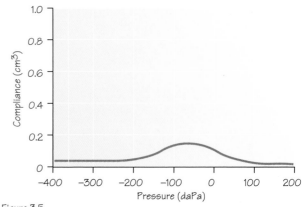

Figure 3.5
A flat tympanometry trace (e.g. in a middle ear effusion/glue ear)

Voice tests and tuning fork tests are easily carried out in a doctor's office with little or no equipment.

Voice tests

A good idea of how well a patient hears can be established through simple observation – can he/she hear normal conversational voice or do you have to raise your voice to make yourself clear? If a patient is deaf, you need to know roughly how much and what type (conductive, sensorineural or mixed) of hearing loss he/she has (see Chapter 4). Simple voice/whisper tests can be conducted for a crude assessment of hearing level.

Tuning fork tests

Tuning fork tests can help with lateralising deafness and with deciding which type of hearing loss is present (Figures 3.1 and 3.2).

TIPS FOR TUNING FORK TESTS

- Use a 512-KHz fork with a good heavy base.
- If the hearing is equal in both ears, the **Weber test** will not lateralise to one side (i.e. the patient will hear the sound in the middle).
- If the Weber is to one side, this can indicate that the other side has little or no hearing, or that there is a conductive deafness on the side the patient identifies as better. Try it yourself – put your finger firmly in the external canal of your own ear and place the tuning fork on your head; you should hear it louder on the side you have blocked as you have given yourself a mild conductive hearing loss.
- The **Rinne test** is negative if the patient hears the sound better by bone conduction. Usually this means there is a conductive loss on that side.
- Be careful interpreting the Rinne test if the patient has profound hearing loss on one side. A Rinne negative may be because he/she hears sound transmitted across the head from a good ear – **false negative Rinne**. Masking of the good ear with a noise box helps overcome this problem.
- Tuning fork tests are quick and easy but skilled audiometry is essential to assess and classify deafness.

Pure tone audiometry

Voice tests and tuning fork tests are helpful, but fairly crude. Formal testing is required for an accurate assessment of hearing levels. For adults and older children who can co-operate (age 4 years upwards), this is best done by pure tone audiometry (PTA).

PTA is performed in a sound-proofed room. The patient is presented with a series of sounds and indicates when he/she can hear them. Air conduction is tested by sounds fed through a headphone; bone conduction by sounds used to vibrate a probe placed on the mastoid bone. The graph is plotted across different frequencies as in Figure 3.3. This is performed separately for each ear.

Evoked response audiometry

PTA needs the patient's co-operation and is therefore a subjective test. To test the hearing objectively a stimulus is presented to the ear and the resultant changes in electrical activity in the nervous system can be measured. These techniques, evoked or electrical response audiometry (ERA), are widely used in children and in disputed cases in adults.

Otoacoustic emissions

Electrical signals are generated by the normal inner ear in response to a sound. These are referred to as 'otoacoustic emissions' (OAE) and are used as a screening test for hearing in newborn children. OAEs will be absent if the child is deaf.

Hearing tests in children

PTA can be very difficult in young children (under 4 years) or in older children and adults with learning difficulties. A skilled tester can use various behavioural audiometry techniques to obtain an accurate assessment of the child's hearing.

Tympanometry

Tympanometry relies on a device that puffs a small current of air into the ear and measures the degree of 'distensibility' of the eardrum and middle ear. A normal trace with a peak (Figure 3.4) suggests that the drum is intact and there is air under normal pressure. A 'flat' tympanogram (Figure 3.5) is typical of a middle ear effusion/glue ear.

Clinical practice point

Always take the parents' concerns about their child's hearing seriously. Early detection of deafness in children may result in a crucial difference to overall outcome.

4 Hearing loss

Figure 4.1
Causes of hearing loss

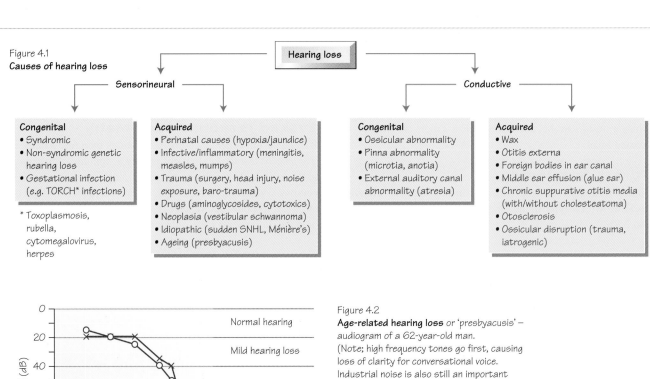

Hearing loss

Sensorineural

Congenital
- Syndromic
- Non-syndromic genetic hearing loss
- Gestational infection (e.g. TORCH* infections)

* Toxoplasmosis, rubella, cytomegalovirus, herpes

Acquired
- Perinatal causes (hypoxia/jaundice)
- Infective/inflammatory (meningitis, measles, mumps)
- Trauma (surgery, head injury, noise exposure, baro-trauma)
- Drugs (aminoglycosides, cytotoxics)
- Neoplasia (vestibular schwannoma)
- Idiopathic (sudden SNHL, Ménière's)
- Ageing (presbyacusis)

Conductive

Congenital
- Ossicular abnormality
- Pinna abnormality (microtia, anotia)
- External auditory canal abnormality (atresia)

Acquired
- Wax
- Otitis externa
- Foreign bodies in ear canal
- Middle ear effusion (glue ear)
- Chronic suppurative otitis media (with/without cholesteatoma)
- Otosclerosis
- Ossicular disruption (trauma, iatrogenic)

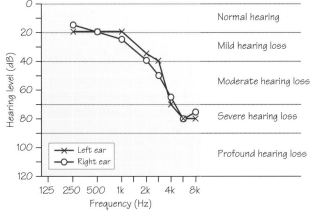

Figure 4.2
Age-related hearing loss or 'presbyacusis' – audiogram of a 62-year-old man.
(Note; high frequency tones go first, causing loss of clarity for conversational voice. Industrial noise is also still an important cause of high tone deafness, especially in men)

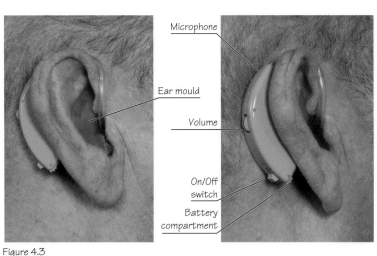

Figure 4.3
Digital hearing aid – 'behind the ear'
A hearing aid amplifies sound. It is only useful for patients with some residual hearing. Hearing aid technology has improved considerably in recent years. Digital aids have predominantly replaced the older analogue models

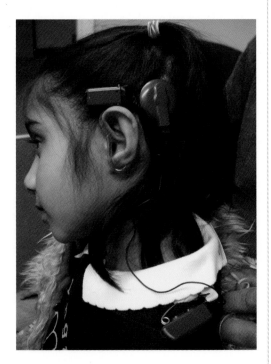

Figure 4.4
Cochlear implant

Ear, Nose and Throat at a Glance, First Edition. Nazia Munir and Ray Clarke.

Epidemiology and classification

The World Health Organization estimates that nearly 300 million people – 5% of the world's population – have a disabling hearing impairment. When classifying the severity of deafness, the hearing level in the better hearing ear is most relevant, as this is the ear the patient relies on.

In developed western countries about 1 in 1000 children is born deaf (congenital deafness). This is much more common in the developing world. The majority of these children have permanent sensorineural loss. This can be part of a syndrome – syndromic deafness (e.g. Usher's syndrome) or it can be an isolated problem that is not part of any definite pattern of anomalies – non-syndromic deafness. More and more cases of non-syndromic deafness are now known to result from a genetic cause (e.g. connexin 22 defects). Early diagnosis of congenital deafness is essential for the best outcome, hence the importance of detecting hearing loss in the newborn infant.

Many people become deaf later in childhood or as they progress through adult life (acquired deafness). Some deterioration in hearing is a part of ageing – presbyacusis (Figure 4.2).

Deafness – as we saw in Chapter 3 – may be conductive or sensorineural. It can be congenital (present at birth) or acquired (comes on after birth, e.g. due to meningitis in infancy). Some of the common causes of each are shown in Figure 4.1.

Sudden sensorineural hearing loss

Sudden unexpected sensorineural deafness is a devastating event. It is defined as a sensorineural hearing loss (SNHL) of at least 30 db or more in three contiguous frequencies over a period of less than 3 days. Incidence is approximately 20 cases per 100,000 per year and peak age of incidence is 50–59 years. It is usually unilateral but may rarely be bilateral.

Sudden SNHL is of unknown aetiology but a number of causes including a vascular event, viral aetiology or breaks in the cochlear membrane may be postulated. Infrequently, identifiable causes such as vestibular schwannoma (acoustic neuroma) are identified.

There is no good evidence that treatment helps but steroids are often given and in some cases spontaneous recovery may occur.

Diagnosis and management

Early diagnosis makes a big difference to the outcome in deaf children. All newborn children in western countries now have their hearing tested (Newborn Hearing Screening Programme) so that late diagnosis has become very rare. This is not the case in the developing world where children still present with deafness at the age of 2, 3 or even older. As soon as it is clear that a child is deaf they should be referred to the Audiology Service for further tests and to commence rehabilitation. A hearing aid can be fitted as early as 2 or 3 weeks after birth.

If the hearing loss is mild or moderate a hearing aid may be all that is needed. Most deaf children can go to mainstream schools, but some are best managed in special schools and 'signing' is still widely used in many parts of the world.

In profoundly deaf children and some adults, an electronic implant – cochlear implant (Figure 4.4) – can help the cochlea respond to sound energy by transmitting it to the brain. Cochlear implants are expensive and not widely available in many parts of the developing world, but have been a great advance in the management of deaf children.

In addition to ENT surgeons, deaf children also require active input from audiological physicians, audiologists, paediatricians, teachers of the deaf, speech and language therapists and, most importantly, parents and siblings. The modes of rehabilitation include:

• Hearing aids (Figure 4.3)
• Special schooling
• Sign language
• Implantable aiding devices (e.g. cochlear implants)

Clinical practice point

Hearing rehabilitation is a multidisciplinary process. Early diagnosis is the key to successful management of the deaf child.

5 The pinna

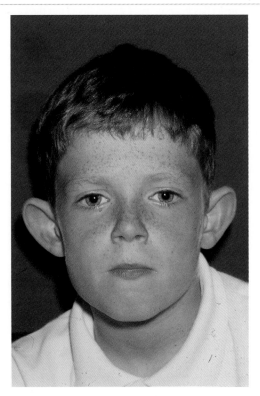

Figure 5.1
Five-year-old boy with prominent ears

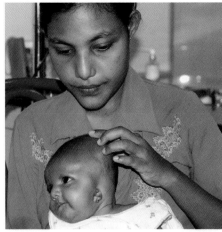
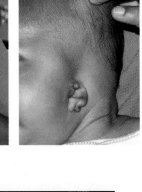

Figure 5.2
Severe microtia

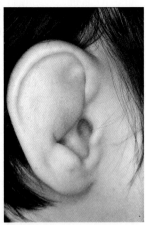

Figure 5.4
Auricular haematoma
A bleed in the space between
the cartilage and the adherent
perichondrium causes blood to
collect under the skin. The ear
is tender and swollen

Pre-auricular sinus

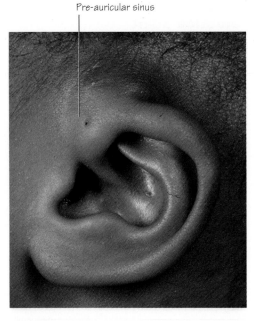

Figure 5.3
Pre-auricular sinus

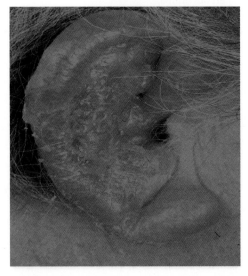

Figure 5.5
Perichondritis

Ear, Nose and Throat at a Glance, First Edition. Nazia Munir and Ray Clarke.

Protruding ears (bat ears)

'Bat ears' are common in children (Figure 5.1). In newborn babies, a specially designed splint (Gault splint®) can help to reform the helical fold. In older children, parents often request surgery around the time the child starts school to minimise teasing and bullying.

Congenital malformations

Microtia Abnormalities of development of the external ear range from minor anomalies to complete absence of the external ear (Figure 5.2). Surgical reconstruction is very challenging. Good quality prostheses are now available but are not usually needed until the child is older. Always make sure the child's hearing is carefully checked. Microtia may be part of a syndrome or one of a series of congenital malformations so the child needs careful examination and investigation by a paediatrician.

Pre-auricular sinus A small sinus in front of the external ear (Figure 5.3) is fairly common and can be removed surgically.

Skin tags are fairly common and can be easily removed if troublesome.

Trauma to the external ear

Penetrating trauma The pinna is exposed at the side of the head and very vulnerable to trauma. Bruises, lacerations and even complete avulsion can occur. Lacerations can be readily repaired with a good aesthetic outcome unless there is severe tissue loss.

Blunt trauma Blunt trauma can cause a bleed between the skin and cartilage – haematoma auris. This can come about after a slap or punch on the ear. If it is not treated promptly the carti- lage can necrose due to pressure, causing an unsightly deformity ('cauliflower ear'). The blood needs to be drained and the layer kept together with a pressure dressing (Figure 5.4).

Inflammation of the pinna

Skin disorders e.g. eczema, erysipelas, psoriasis and infected hair follicles (furunculosis) can involve the external ear.

Diffuse otitis externa Infection in the ear canal (otitis externa; see Chapter 8) can spread to the pinna. If the infection is severe it may involve the cartilage (perichondritis), causing red painful swelling (Figure 5.5).

Tumours of the external ear

Benign swellings These include painful deposits on the rim of the pinna in gout (gouty tophus). The painful nodules elderly men sometimes get at the tip of the helix are due to small vascular tumours – chondrodermatitis nodularis.

Malignant tumours The pinna is exposed to a lot of sunlight and is a common site for the development of both basal cell carcinoma (BCC) and squamous cell carcinoma (SCC). White-skinned people – particularly elderly men – who work outdoors are especially at risk. These cancers are usually localised; the prognosis is excellent if they are treated early.

Clinical practice points

- Auricular haematoma should be drained early to avoid cartilage necrosis.
- A neoplastic diagnosis should always be considered in patients with ulcerating lesions of the pinna.

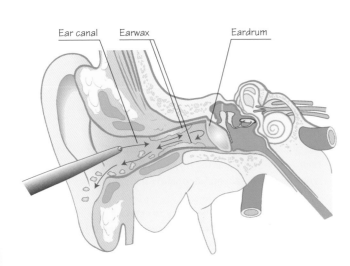

Ear canal   Earwax   Eardrum

Figure 6.1
Ear syringing
This can be performed by a trained doctor or nurse.
The tip of a water-filled syringe is placed just inside
the ear canal, and a stream of warm water is gently
directed into the canal to remove earwax or a foreign
body by pushing it out of the ear canal

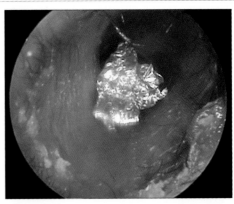

Figure 6.2a
A piece of foil in the external auditory canal

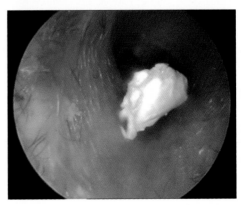

Figure 6.2b
A piece of polystyrene in the external auditory canal

Earwax

Wax or cerumen is normal. It is made of a mixture of keratin (shed skin) with viscous (oily) secretions from sebaceous glands and from modified apocrine (sweat) glands. The migrates out from the eardrum. If it becomes impacted it can cause deafness. Patients – and particularly parents – need to be advised not to poke hairclips, pens, tissue paper or spectacle frames in the ear. The ear is self-cleansing. Meddling with it only causes the wax to become impacted and may traumatise the ear canal causing otitis externa.

If wax does impact and needs to be removed this should be painless and straightforward. If you have access to a microscope and good quality instruments for removing wax under direct vision this is ideal, otherwise wax is best dealt with by gentle syringing (Figure 6.1).

Foreign bodies

Children, and occasionally adults, put objects such as beads, cotton buds, pieces of sponge and crayons in their ears (Figure 6.2). They can cause otitis externa and are best removed. Gentle syringing may help but sometimes the child needs a general anaesthetic for removal. It is easy to push a foreign body further in. Try to use an instrument that helps secure the foreign body and above all be gentle. Caution should be exercised with button batteries as they can leak and quickly cause severe corrosion of the skin and need to be removed as an emergency.

TIPS FOR EAR SYRINGING

- Take a good history. If the patient has a perforated eardrum, syringing is best avoided.
- Check the ear canal with an otoscope to make sure there is no active infection.
- If the wax is hard and does not easily come away, prescribe warm olive oil or ceruminolytic drops for a few days to soften it.
- Make sure you have a good light.
- Protect the patient's clothing with towels. Syringing can be messy!
- Clean tap water is fine but make sure it is at body temperature.
- Direct the stream toward the roof of the ear canal. If a high stream is directed at the drum it can cause a perforation.

Clinical practice points

- Wax is normal. It only needs to be removed if it has become impacted or is infected.
- Corrosive material – such as batteries – in the ear canal need to be removed urgently.

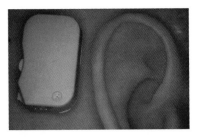

Figure 7.1
A bone-anchored hearing aid

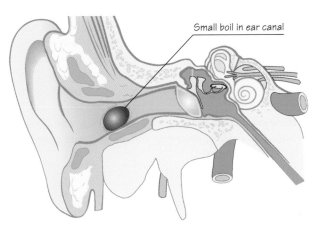

Small boil in ear canal

Figure 7.2
A furuncle (boil) in the ear canal
This is extremely painful

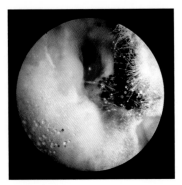

Figure 7.3
Otomycosis
Note the fungal hyphae

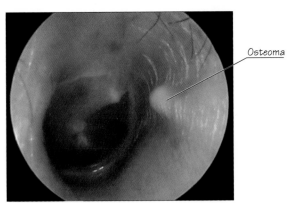

Osteoma

Figure 7.5
A very small osteoma in the right ear canal

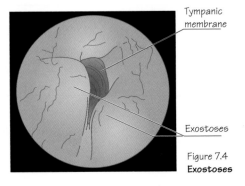

Tympanic
membrane

Exostoses

Figure 7.4
Exostoses

Ear, Nose and Throat at a Glance, First Edition. Nazia Munir and Ray Clarke.

The external auditory canal (ear canal) is lined with hair-bearing skin and is part of the external ear (see Chapter 1).

Congenital anomalies

The external ear canal may be poorly developed or even absent. This can be an isolated anomaly, but it is more often part of a significant deformity of the external ear, sometimes involving the middle ear and rarely the inner ear (microtia; see Chapter 5). The child may also be deaf and management can be very difficult as a conventional hearing aid will not fit in the ear canal. If the child has some inner ear (cochlear) hearing function he/she may need a bone anchored hearing aid (BAHA). This is fitted behind the ear on to a titanium screw which is attached to the skull (Figure 7.1).

Inflammation and infection

The skin of the external ear is sensitive and can be exposed to water, pathogens and trauma from, for example, hair clips and cotton buds which many patients and parents will use to clean the ear canals and to attempt to remove wax. The main clinical features of inflammation of the external ear are pain, itching and discharge.

Skin disorders Eczema, psoriasis and skin allergies may all involve the external ear canals. The treatment is that of the underlying disorder, but applying topical treatment to the inflamed external ear canal can be difficult because of pain and swelling.

Otitis externa The skin of the ear canal is prone to infection (otitis externa). This is sometimes known as 'swimmer's ear' as one important aetiological factor is infection of the ear canal following swimming. When the skin of the ear canal becomes macerated, or is traumatised by, for example, a cotton bud, bacterial infection can supervene. Common organisms include *Pseudomonas* spp. and *Staphylococcus* spp. The patient will have pain, itching and sometimes a smelly discharge. The treatment is to clean out the ear, keep it dry and use a short course of antibiotic drops. Drops containing a combination of antibiotics and steroids may be used to help tackle both the infection and the inflammatory changes simultaneously. Severe cases may need regular aural toilet with microsuction at an ENT clinic. Excessive and prolonged use of antibiotics can alter the flora of the external ear. This can give rise to even more problematic infection including fungal infection (otomycosis).

Furunculosis Infection of the hair follicle in the external ear can cause a localised swelling – furuncle (Figure 7.2). This is extremely tender and painful. It is often caused by *Staphylococcus* spp. Severe cases are best treated by puncturing the furuncle to drain the pus under aseptic conditions. The patient will then need topical treatment for several days.

Otomycosis (Figure 7.3) Fungal infection of the ear canal often takes hold in a patient who has a long-standing ear infection particularly if he/she has had frequent and prolonged treatment with antibiotic drops. Often, the fungal hyphae are easily evident on looking at the ear canal. The patient will have severe itching. The best treatment is to perform regular aural toilet with microsuction and to use anti-fungal drops (e.g. clotrimazole) often for several weeks.

Tumours
Exostoses and osteomas

True neoplasms are very rare. Bony swellings – exostoses and osteomas – are more common. Exostoses are broad-based and often bilateral. They arise from the anterior and posterior canal walls and are often found in cold water swimmers where they are thought to represent an inflammatory response to extremes of temperature (Figure 7.4). Wax can collect behind exostoses and if they are very large and symptomatic they may need to be removed surgically.

Osteomas (Figure 7.5) are benign bony tumours of the ear canal. They are more prevalent in males and tend to be unilateral and form discrete, pedunculated masses arising from the area of the junction of bony and cartilaginous ear canal. There is no association with cold water exposure. If they are very large and become symptomatic they may need to be removed surgically.

Malignant/necrotising otitis externa

Malignant/necrotising otitis externa is an aggressive condition. The term 'malignant' is a misnomer as the condition is not neoplastic but rather a progressive osteomyelitis of the temporal bone resulting from otitis externa. Patients with compromised immunity (e.g. poorly controlled diabetics) are particularly at risk. The main presenting complaint is severe, unremitting, deep-seated pain that is not responsive to analgesics. Clinical examination may reveal findings consistent with a simple otitis externa or in severe cases florid granulations arising from the osteitic bone may be evident. A high index of suspicion in high-risk patients is required. Regular aural toilet, systemic and topical antibiotics and in some cases surgical débridement of the involved bone may be required. If untreated this condition has a high morbidity and mortality.

Clinical practice point

Otitis externa can be prolonged and painful. Gentle but thorough removal of debris from the ear canal hastens resolution.

8 Acute otitis media

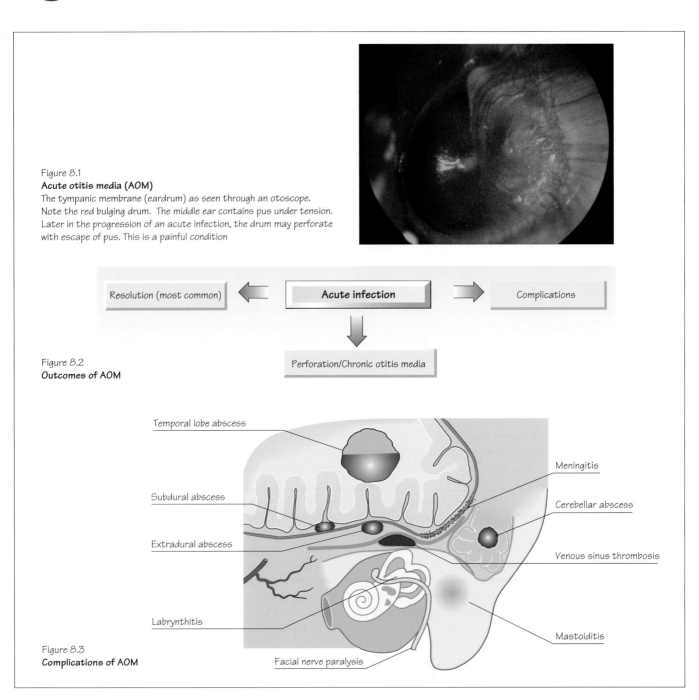

Figure 8.1
Acute otitis media (AOM)
The tympanic membrane (eardrum) as seen through an otoscope.
Note the red bulging drum. The middle ear contains pus under tension.
Later in the progression of an acute infection, the drum may perforate
with escape of pus. This is a painful condition

Resolution (most common) ← **Acute infection** → Complications

Perforation/Chronic otitis media

Figure 8.2
Outcomes of AOM

Temporal lobe abscess
Meningitis
Subdural abscess
Cerebellar abscess
Extradural abscess
Venous sinus thrombosis
Labrynthitis
Mastoiditis
Facial nerve paralysis

Figure 8.3
Complications of AOM

Acute otitis media

Acute otitis media (AOM) is inflammation (usually caused by infection) of the middle ear (Figure 8.1). It is the most common infection seen in children. About 90% of children will have had one or more episodes of acute otitis media by their second birthday. Infection is usually initially with a virus and comes from the nose or pharynx ascending via the Eustachian tube. AOM does occur in adults, but much less often. The Eustachian tube in children is shorter, wider and more horizontal than in adults, so that infection tracks upwards much more easily. Additionally, children are also more susceptible to infections in general because of their immature defence mechanisms. Adults may develop otitis media but much less frequently.

The usual organisms are viruses and the 'pyogenic' bacteria (e.g. streptococci, *Haemophilus influenzae*).

Clinical presentation

The main clinical features of AOM are **otalgia** (earache), **fever** and **deafness** followed by **otorrhoea** (discharge from the ear, often sticky; if infected with anaerobic organism it may be fetid).

The child is usually fractious and has a pyrexia. Older children may complain of earache, but babies may not be able to localise pain. Parents usually say the pain is much worse at night and keeps the child awake. Viral infection is short-lived, but bacterial infection can last for a week or more. The middle ear fills with pus causing the eardrum to bulge. This is intensely painful, but often the pain is relieved as the eardrum bursts and the parents notice a discharge. Often, there is residual fluid in the middle ear for several weeks after an AOM and the child is a little deaf. Diagnosis is made by taking a careful history and examination. It can be difficult to obtain a good view of the eardrum particularly in a young child. Figure 8.2 shows the typical outcomes of AOM.

Infection in the middle ear will always spread to the mastoid to some degree and in severe cases otitis media can be complicated by a mastoid abscess. The mastoid bone behind the ear is tender and swollen and if infection spreads beyond the bone an abscess can develop in the skin around the mastoid. Otitis media can also spread to the inner ear, the facial nerve and the brain (Figure 8.3).

Treatment and prognosis

Most cases of AOM resolve without any adverse effects. Complications, when they occur, can be serious and even life-threatening. Antibiotic treatment of AOM is controversial. Many authorities feel that for short-lived infections analgesia is all that is required, as the organism is usually a virus. Even bacterial infections do not seem to be influenced greatly by antibiotics, which at best hasten resolution by a day or so. However, if a child has a serious bacterial AOM that has not resolved over 24 hours then it is sensible to prescribe a cephalosporin or amoxicillin. It is most important to manage the child's pain. Very rarely, if symptoms persist – and certainly if complications have developed – the child may need a drainage operation to remove pus from the middle ear (paracentesis, or a myringotomy). Mastoiditis and intracranial sepsis will require specialised surgery.

In summary, the management of AOM consists of:
• Analgesia
• Antibiotics – not always needed
• Surgery for complications – rarely required

Clinical practice points

• The most important symptom to control in AOM is pain. Give strong and frequent analgesics (e.g. paracetamol and non-steroidal analgesics).
• If there are complications the child needs urgent hospital admission.

9 Perforated eardrum

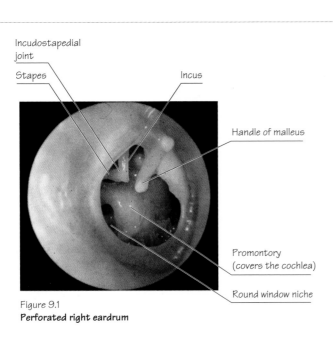

- Incudostapedial joint
- Stapes
- Incus
- Handle of malleus
- Promontory (covers the cochlea)
- Round window niche

Figure 9.1
Perforated right eardrum

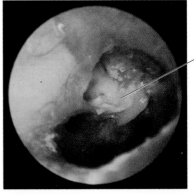

- Squamous epithelium (cholesteatoma)

Figure 9.2
Cholesteatoma
This is erosive and may eventually give rise to intracranial complications

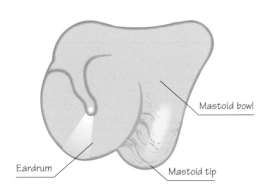

- Mastoid bowl
- Eardrum
- Mastoid tip

Figure 9.3
Mastoid cavity (left ear)

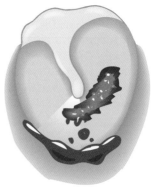

Figure 9.4
Traumatic perforation of the left drum

Ear, Nose and Throat at a Glance, First Edition. Nazia Munir and Ray Clarke.
© 2013 Nazia Munir and Ray Clarke. Published 2013 by Blackwell Publishing Ltd.

Chronic suppurative otitis media

Acute otitis media can lead to the infection rupturing the eardrum, leaving a perforation (Figure 9.1). This usually heals, but may persist and cause recurrent episodes of discharge (chronic suppurative otitis media, CSOM).

In addition to discharge, the patient may complain of increasing deafness. Persistent infections can lead to spread of infection beyond the ear, resulting in intracranial or extracranial complications (see Chapter 8).

Presentation

A perforation of the eardrum may cause little or no trouble. The ear is liable to discharge when the patient has a respiratory tract infection or if the ear gets wet (e.g. after swimming or hair washing). Some degree of hearing loss is inevitable but it may be slight. If in addition to the perforation the infection has eroded the ossicles, deafness can be more severe. The cochlea is usually not involved so hearing loss is conductive and incomplete.

Treatment of a perforated eardrum

Management options include the following:
• *Conservative management.* If a perforation is asymptomatic, simple reassurance and advice regarding water precautions is all that is required.
• *Topical antibiotic drops.* In patients with intermittent episodes of discharge short courses of topical antibiotic drops, in addition to water precautions, may be all that is needed to keep things under control. Many of the available preparations contain aminoglycosides and may be toxic to the inner ear, especially with prolonged use. Consider ciprofloxacin if a prolonged course of treatment is required, to reduce the risk of ototoxicity.
• *Myringoplasty.* In cases of recurrent discharge or if the patient wants surgical intervention (e.g. to enable him/her to swim) the eardrum defect can be repaired surgically (myringoplasty). The procedure involves placing a graft (e.g. temporalis fascia, taken from behind the ear) under the eardrum remnant allowing the epithelium to re-grow and close the defect.

Cholesteatoma

In severe cases, squamous epithelium from the skin of the external ear migrates into the middle ear and collects in a mass (Figure 9.2), which can become erosive and gradually eats away at bone and soft tissue, making spread of infection into the brain, the inner ear and the facial nerve more likely. Cholesteatoma is a serious condition and patients need to be referred to an ENT surgeon for assessment and probable surgery. Cholesteatoma should be suspected if there is a perforated eardrum with:
• Persistent smelly discharge
• No improvement with drops
• Severe hearing loss
• Dizziness
• Unexplained neurological symptoms or signs.

Cholesteatoma can result in serious complications if left untreated:
• Progressive hearing loss
• Acute mastoiditis
• Labyrinthitis
• Facial palsy
• Meningitis
• Intracranial abscesses
• Venous sinus thrombosis.

Treatment of cholesteatoma requires surgical input. All the diseased tissue has to be removed and usually it is necessary to drill away much of the diseased bone in the mastoid. The procedure is referred to as a mastoidectomy (Figure 9.3).

Trauma to the middle ear

Occasionally, the eardrum can be perforated by an injury – either sharp trauma or a blow to the side of the head (Figure 9.4). Usually, this will heal itself. Blunt trauma to the middle ear can cause a bleed behind an intact eardrum (haemotympanum). This causes a conductive deafness – usually temporary – and is typically short-lived, resolving without the need for intervention.

Clinical practice point

If there is any suspicion of a cholesteatoma in a perforated eardrum refer the patient for an ENT opinion.

10 Otitis media with effusion

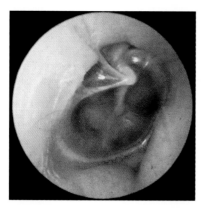

Figure 10.1
Otoscopic view of the eardrum in otitis media with effusion (OME)
Note the retracted, translucent drum. The middle ear is filled with a sticky 'glue-like' fluid

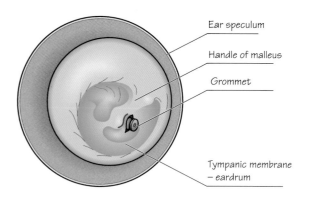

Ear speculum

Handle of malleus

Grommet

Tympanic membrane – eardrum

Figure 10.2
A grommet acts as a two-way conduit to allow air into the middle ear. It is inserted in a small, surgically created hole (myringotomy) in the eardrum

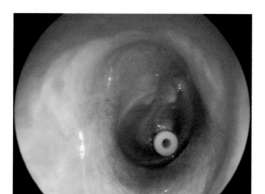

Figure 10.3
A grommet in position

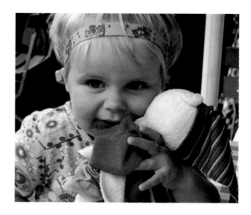

Figure 10.4
Child using a Softband™
Many children (and parents) will prefer to avoid grommets and use a hearing aid instead. Another approach is to use a Softband™. A small microphone is attached to this band and picks up and amplifies sound

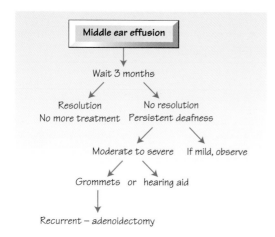

Middle ear effusion

Wait 3 months

Resolution
No more treatment

No resolution
Persistent deafness

Moderate to severe

If mild, observe

Grommets or hearing aid

Recurrent – adenoidectomy

Figure 10.5
Evidence-based management of OME

Definition

Otitis media with effusion (OME) is the persistence of fluid in the middle ear for a period of 3 months or more. It is also referred to as 'glue ear'.

Incidence and aetiology

OME is the most common cause of hearing loss in children. Persistent fluid in the middle ear is common following an episode of acute otitis media (AOM). Most parents will notice that children may be slightly deaf for several weeks after an ear infection. Fluid persisting for more than 3 months is pathological and is termed OME.

The prevalence of OME is highest in children from the age of about 2 to 7 years. Up to 30% of children in this age group at any one time may be affected. OME is more prevalent in winter than summer months. It may be caused by infection, but pressure changes in the middle ear associated with Eustachian tube dysfunction are also implicated. The adenoids can have an important role, either because of infection spreading from the adenoids into the ear via the Eustachian tube or because they contribute to Eustachian tube obstruction and pressure changes in the middle ear. Another theory is that the adenoids become coated with a matrix (biofilm) that is resistant to the immune defences and to antibiotics and contributes to recurrent infections in the ear mucosa. Children with Down syndrome and cleft palate are especially susceptible to OME.

Effects

Children with OME have a mild to moderate conductive hearing loss. If this is unilateral it causes little if any trouble; if it is bilateral and persistent the child may start to struggle in school. The parents will often notice that the child turns the television up loud and in prolonged cases OME can interfere with the development of speech. Children may also have mild episodes of dizziness and clumsiness. Unless they also have AOM they will not usually have pain. Some children may develop behavioural problems as a result of hearing loss associated with OME.

Presentation and diagnosis

Take a careful history enquiring about the child's general and speech development and school performance and how he/she responds to ordinary conversation at home. The changes on inspecting the eardrum can be subtle, but sometimes you will see a fluid level or a translucent eardrum resulting from accumulated sticky fluid (Figure 10.1).

Management

Management is initially expectant (i.e. wait and see; Figure 10.5). The condition resolves in most cases over a period of months. Parents and teachers can help with simple measures such as:
- Getting the child's attention before speaking to him/her
- Facing the child directly when speaking
- Speaking clearly and without mumbling or muttering
- Making sure there is minimum interference from background noise (e.g. televisions).

If deafness persists the most common treatment options include use of a hearing aid device or the insertion of a grommet (Figures 10.2–10.4).

As the condition resolves spontaneously over time the aim of treatment is to help the child's hearing during the period when he/she has an effusion. For this reason many experts now recommend the use of a hearing aid as a temporary measure until the fluid resolves. This can often be over a period of a year or more, and some children and parents may be reluctant to use a hearing aid for this length of time and therefore opt for surgical intervention.

Grommet insertion is performed under a general anaesthetic, usually as a day case. The fluid is aspirated from the middle ear and the grommet helps with re-ventilation of the middle ear. Improvement in hearing is usually immediate. The grommet extrudes over a period of 9 months to a year.

Adenoidectomy can be helpful in severe or recurrent cases.

It is important to reassure parents that OME is a common condition and that it will not affect the child's hearing in the long term.

Clinical practice point

Most middle ear effusions resolve. Reserve treatment for those with a prolonged history and bilateral effusions that have caused significant deafness.

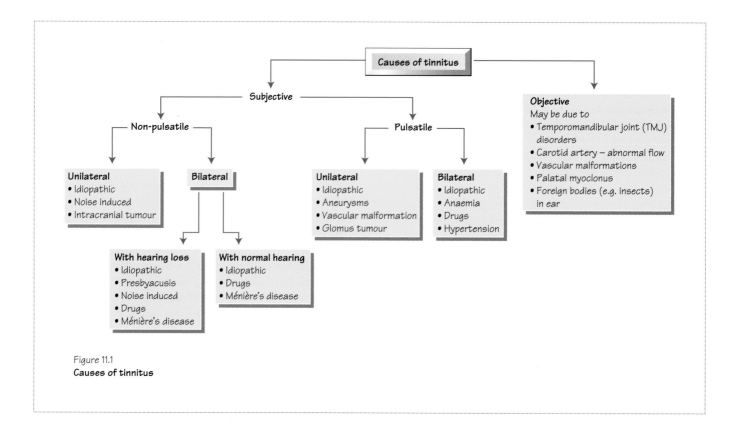

Figure 11.1
Causes of tinnitus

Definition

Tinnitus is noise in the ear or head in the absence of a sound stimulus.

Incidence

Almost everybody experiences tinnitus or noises in the ear at some time or another. It is usually short-lived and may follow exposure to loud noise. It is most noticeable in quiet surroundings and only becomes problematic when it is prolonged and persistent.

Most tinnitus is subjective (heard only by the patient); however, it can be objective (can be heard by an observer). It is usually bilateral and sometimes pulsatile – in time with the heartbeat – in which case it is often caused by rapid blood flow through the vessels of the head and neck. Figure 11.1 demonstrates some of the causes of tinnitus.

Aetiology

In the vast majority of cases the cause of tinnitus is unknown. It is thought to arise because of electrical impulses occurring in the hair cells of the cochlea or inner ear in the absence of an appropriate sound stimulus. This sometimes comes about at an early stage in the development of degenerative disease of the cochlea.

In patients with presbycusis (age-related hearing loss) the deafness may sometimes be preceded by tinnitus. Patients with prolonged exposure to industrial noise will also often complain of tinnitus.

Unilateral tinnitus can very rarely be the presentation of an intracranial tumour and warrants more urgent investigation than bilateral tinnitus for this reason. However, abnormal findings in a patient with tinnitus are uncommon unless there is some other evidence of disease.

Effects on the patient

The effects of tinnitus on the patient vary from mild nuisance to severe distress causing depression and sometimes making the patient contemplate suicide. It is far more troublesome in quiet environments. Patients will often rely on various tricks of their own to lessen the adverse effects. If tinnitus is associated with a moderate or profound hearing loss the effect on the patient's lifestyle can be devastating.

Many patients learn to adapt to tinnitus with time (habituation) and most patients can be reassured that the symptoms do lessen in severity over months.

Investigations

Make sure you take a thorough history from all patients with tinnitus. Enquire in particular about drugs (e.g. asprin is well known to cause tinnitus and many commonly used medicines have tinnitus as a recognised side effect). Enquire about other symptoms, particularly deafness and balance problems, and make sure you carry out a thorough physical examination. This includes measuring the patient's blood pressure and checking for conditions such as anaemia and jaundice. If the tinnitus is pulsatile it may well be caused by systemic or cardiovascular disease. Pulsatile unilateral tinnitus may be idiopathic, but it is important to exclude conditions such as intracranial aneurysms and vascular malformations or the very rare vascular tumours (e.g. glomus tumours) that occur in the middle ear. The patient may need to be referred to an ENT department for audiometry, a computed tomography (CT) or magnetic resonance imaging (MRI) scan.

Management

The management of tinnitus is largely supportive (see box), centred on symptom control. After serious causes of tinnitus have been excluded most patients only require simple reassurance. If there is an associated hearing loss a hearing aid will often help not only the patient's hearing, but also improve the tinnitus.

Clinical practice points

- Tinnitus is a very distressing symptom – treat it seriously.
- Beware so-called miracle cures for tinnitus – they rarely help for long.

A number of devices rely on the principle that tinnitus is much more tolerable in the presence of background noise. Many patients use a 'white noise generator' which fits in and behind the ear much the same as a hearing aid and emits a low-intensity noise that makes the tinnitus much easier to tolerate. Some patients find the use of a radio at night or a small noise fitting device under the pillow (pillow masker) helpful.

Patients who are severely psychologically distressed will need intensive counselling and psychological support (hearing/tinnitus therapy). Drugs are very rarely helpful in the management of tinnitus.

It is helpful for patients to know that this is a common problem and they may appreciate getting in touch with other patients – for example, via the British Tinnitus Association website (www.tinnitus.org.uk).

12 Physiology of balance

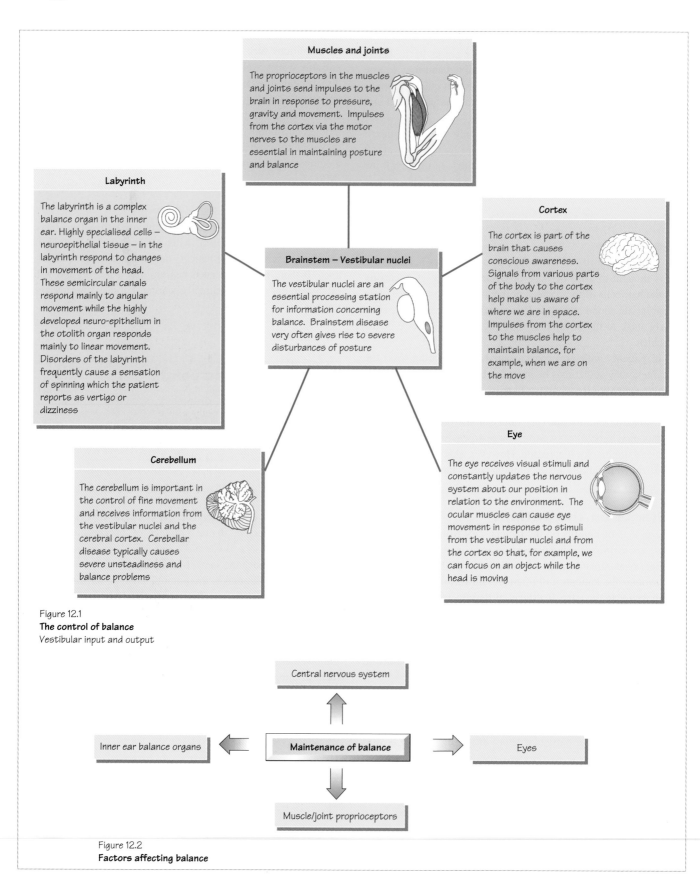

Muscles and joints

The proprioceptors in the muscles and joints send impulses to the brain in response to pressure, gravity and movement. Impulses from the cortex via the motor nerves to the muscles are essential in maintaining posture and balance

Labyrinth

The labyrinth is a complex balance organ in the inner ear. Highly specialised cells – neuroepithelial tissue – in the labyrinth respond to changes in movement of the head. These semicircular canals respond mainly to angular movement while the highly developed neuro-epithelium in the otolith organ responds mainly to linear movement. Disorders of the labyrinth frequently cause a sensation of spinning which the patient reports as vertigo or dizziness

Brainstem – Vestibular nuclei

The vestibular nuclei are an essential processing station for information concerning balance. Brainstem disease very often gives rise to severe disturbances of posture

Cortex

The cortex is part of the brain that causes conscious awareness. Signals from various parts of the body to the cortex help make us aware of where we are in space. Impulses from the cortex to the muscles help to maintain balance, for example, when we are on the move

Cerebellum

The cerebellum is important in the control of fine movement and receives information from the vestibular nuclei and the cerebral cortex. Cerebellar disease typically causes severe unsteadiness and balance problems

Eye

The eye receives visual stimuli and constantly updates the nervous system about our position in relation to the environment. The ocular muscles can cause eye movement in response to stimuli from the vestibular nuclei and from the cortex so that, for example, we can focus on an object while the head is moving

Figure 12.1
The control of balance
Vestibular input and output

Central nervous system

Inner ear balance organs ← **Maintenance of balance** → Eyes

Muscle/joint proprioceptors

Figure 12.2
Factors affecting balance

Ear, Nose and Throat at a Glance, First Edition. Nazia Munir and Ray Clarke.

Physiology of balance

Maintaining balance is a complex physiological process. When it goes wrong, patients may experience dizziness, unsteadiness, falls or 'vertigo' (Figures 12.1 and 12.2).

The vestibular nuclei in the brainstem are a relay station for information from various parts of the body about balance. Nervous connections from the brainstem then send signals to other parts of the nervous system. The eyes, skeletal muscles and the cerebral cortex all respond quickly to changes in posture, head position and body movement and keep us steady on our feet. It is not surprising then that this very sophisticated system can easily fail, especially in elderly patients.

Clinical practice point

The complexity of the physiological process that controls balance helps to explain why so many disorders can have 'disequilibrium' or 'dizziness' as part of their presentation.

See Chapter 13.

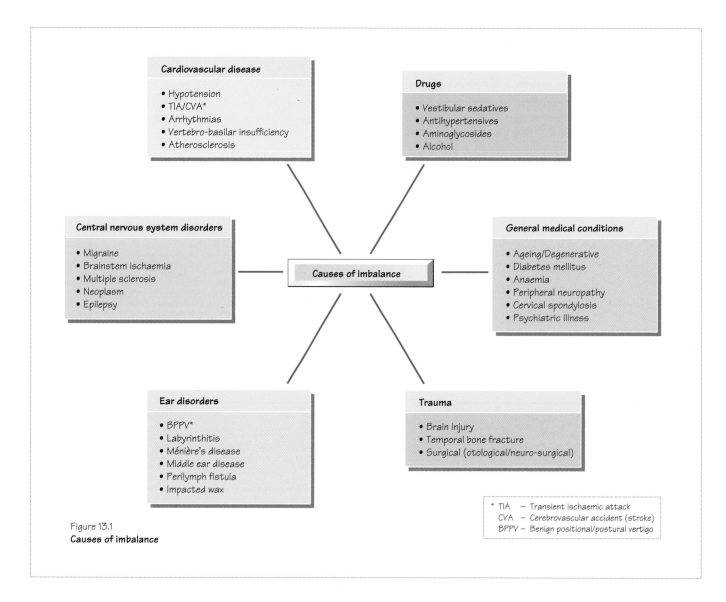

Cardiovascular disease

- Hypotension
- TIA/CVA*
- Arrhythmias
- Vertebro-basilar insufficiency
- Atherosclerosis

Drugs

- Vestibular sedatives
- Antihypertensives
- Aminoglycosides
- Alcohol

Central nervous system disorders

- Migraine
- Brainstem ischaemia
- Multiple sclerosis
- Neoplasm
- Epilepsy

Causes of imbalance

General medical conditions

- Ageing/Degenerative
- Diabetes mellitus
- Anaemia
- Peripheral neuropathy
- Cervical spondylosis
- Psychiatric illness

Ear disorders

- BPPV*
- Labyrinthitis
- Ménière's disease
- Middle ear disease
- Perilymph fistula
- Impacted wax

Trauma

- Brain injury
- Temporal bone fracture
- Surgical (otological/neuro-surgical)

* TIA — Transient ischaemic attack
  CVA — Cerebrovascular accident (stroke)
  BPPV — Benign positional/postural vertigo

Figure 13.1
Causes of imbalance

Ear, Nose and Throat at a Glance, First Edition. Nazia Munir and Ray Clarke.

Table 13.1 Common otological causes of vertigo.

Diagnosis	Symptoms	Features	Management
BPPV	Dizziness Transient nausea	Sudden attacks often precipitated by head movement Short-lived (seconds) Nystagmus	Reassurance Epley manoeuvre Vestibular exercises
Acute labyrinthitis	Dizziness Deafness Nausea	Vomiting Nystagmus Lasts days	Bed rest Vestibular sedatives (short course) Vestibular exercises
Ménière's disease	Deafness Dizziness Tinnitus Aural fullness	Episodic attacks Lasts minutes to hours Vomiting (sometimes) May be nystagmus	Rest Dietary modifications Drugs (betahistine, diuretics, vestibular sedatives p.r.n.) Surgery last resort Vestibular exercises
Middle ear disease (chronic suppurative otitis media)	Deafness Dizziness Otorrhoea Otalgia	Progressive symptoms Foul-smelling discharge Neurological symptoms	Early ENT referral for investigation and management Often need surgery

BPPV, benign paroxysmal positional vertigo; p.r.n., pro re nata (as necessary).

Diagnosing the cause of balance disorders can be challenging. Often – especially in elderly patients – there may be more than one pathology in more than one system.

Vertigo is a hallucination of movement produced by an underlying disorder of the vestibular system. The disturbance may be **peripheral** (in the ear, otological) or **central** (central nervous system). There are many systems that contribute to and are crucial to the control and maintenance of balance. If any one of these systems is affected this can result in the patient experiencing a balance disorder. Some of the conditions that can contribute to balance disorders are shown in Figure 13.1.

Presentation

Good history taking is the main diagnostic tool for diagnosing the underlying origin of a balance disorder. Patients will use various terms to describe imbalance, e.g. 'dizzy spells', 'funny turns' and 'vertigo'. It is important to differentiate between the following and establish exactly what the patient is describing:
• *Vertigo*: hallucination of movement (due to vestibular disorders)
• *Light headedness*: feeling faint (often due to cardiovascular disturbance)
• *Unsteadiness*: problems with gait (may be age related or due to central nervous system disorders)
• *Blackouts*: loss of consciousness (may be cardiovascular or neurological in origin).

Vertigo is often rotatory and the patient describes a spinning sensation. Some will describe it like the feeling that they get after going on a merry-go-round ride.

Once the presence of vertigo has been established ascertain the following:
• Onset and duration of the first attack
• Associated otological symptoms: tinnitus, hearing change, otalgia, otorrhoea
• Associated non-otological symptoms: nausea, vomiting, fever, systemic upset, preceding viral illness

• Exacerbating and relieving factors: effects of change in posture, head/neck movement, effect of darkness
• Co-morbidities: general health, cardiovascular/neurological/psychological conditions, diabetes
• Drug history
• Social history: alcohol intake, recreational drug use
• Family history: migraine, degenerative diseases.

Examination

Assess for abnormality of gait as the patient walks into the consultation room. A full ear examination including otoscopy, tuning fork tests, pure tone audiometry and tympanometry where appropriate is needed in patients experiencing vertigo.

Full cranial nerve examination, cerebellar function testing and testing the eyes for nystagmus are also pertinent. Positional testing (Dix–Hallpike test) is also mandatory in the balance clinic.

Otological causes of vertigo

In most cases of acute vertigo the initial management is expectant and supportive, with bed rest and a short course of vestibular sedatives where required. Prolonged use of vestibular sedatives should be avoided and actively discouraged as this can severely compromise recovery. Table 13.1 shows the presenting symptoms, features and management of some of the more common otological causes of vertigo.

Early input from vestibular physiotherapists can be invaluable for patients with balance disorders.

Clinical practice point

Prolonged use of vestibular sedatives should be avoided and actively discouraged in patients with vertigo of any cause, as this can severely compromise recovery.

See Chapter 12.

14 The facial nerve

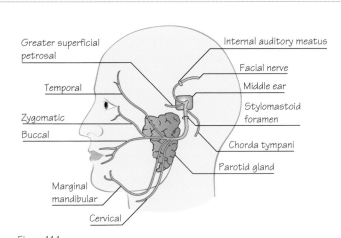

Figure 14.1
The branches of the facial nerve

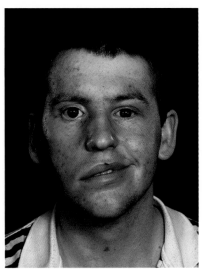

Figure 14.3
38-year-old man with right facial palsy

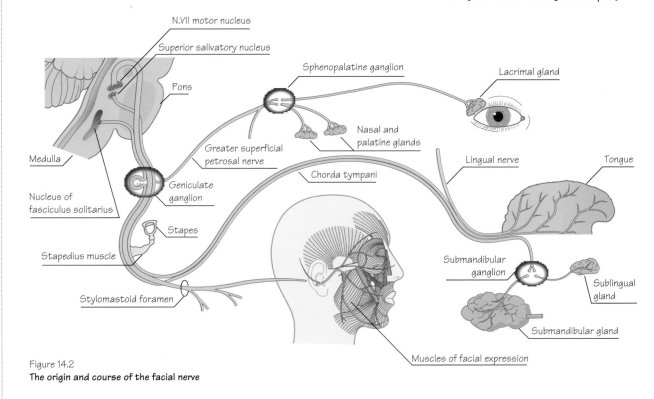

Figure 14.2
The origin and course of the facial nerve

Ear, Nose and Throat at a Glance, First Edition. Nazia Munir and Ray Clarke.

Applied anatomy

The facial nerve (Figures 14.1 and 14.2) is the motor nerve to the muscles of facial expression. Smiling, frowning and expressing emotions are dependent on its normal function. It begins in the facial nucleus in the brainstem (the pons), passes close to the internal auditory meatus to run in the middle ear and mastoid and then exits the skull at the stylomastoid foramen just in front of the mastoid process. It then runs in the parotid gland. It breaks into two divisions, the zygomatic-temporal and the mandibulo-cervical, which between them have five branches (Figure 14.1) supplying the muscles of facial expression.

The nerve has a long course and is vulnerable to injury at several sites (Figure 14.2). Facial paralysis (Figure 14.3) can be a devastating condition for the patient.

Facial palsy

A patient suffering stroke will often have a facial palsy but the forehead muscles are spared as they have innervations from both sides (supranuclear/upper motor neurone palsy). If the nerve is injured below the pons (infranuclear/lower motor neurone palsy), the paralysis can be complete and involves the forehead and the facial muscles.

The patient will have weakness of the muscles on one side, difficulty closing the eye and clearing the cheek after eating, and sometimes drooling from one side of the mouth. Taste and the production of tears can be affected. The extent of weakness is variable and the palsy may be partial or complete.

Causes of facial palsy

Pathology can affect the facial nerve anywhere from its origin in the brainstem to the peripheral branches. Many cases are of unknown origin – 'idiopathic'. This is also known as Bell's palsy. It is important to exclude other causes before making the diagnosis of Bell's palsy. A full history and examination are paramount. Patients with persistent facial palsy that does not resolve will need to be referred for investigation.

Causes of facial palsy

- Stroke (upper motor neurone palsy)
- Ear disease (e.g. cholesteatoma, malignancy)
- Parotid lesions
- Trauma (e.g. head injury, iatrogenic injury)
- Infection (e.g. herpes zoster, acute otitis media, malignant/necrotising otitis externa)
- Idiopathic (Bell's palsy)

Management of facial paralysis

The treatment is dependent on the cause of facial paralysis. Bell's palsy (i.e. unknown cause) is the most common presentation of lower motor neurone facial palsy. High dose steroids over a short period are often prescribed in Bell's palsy. The evidence is inconclusive, but if steroids are going to be used it is important to use them as soon as possible after the onset of symptoms. Anti-viral drugs are also sometimes used on the basis that Bell's palsy is probably caused by a viral infection. Once again the evidence is inconclusive. Surgery is very rarely required.

The most crucial aspect of management is to ensure good eye care and protection. The eye is at risk of conjunctivitis and corneal erosions. If the eye cannot be completely closed, taping the eye shut when the patient is asleep is a useful initial measure alongside regular use of lubricating eye drops.

Management of facial paralysis

- Exclude identifiable causes of paralysis
- Protect the eye
- Steroids
- Aciclovir
- Surgery rarely needed (decompression)

Clinical practice point

Bell's palsy is a diagnosis of exclusion. Always check for other causes. If a facial palsy persists arrange urgent assessment.

---

15 The nose and paranasal sinuses: applied anatomy and examination

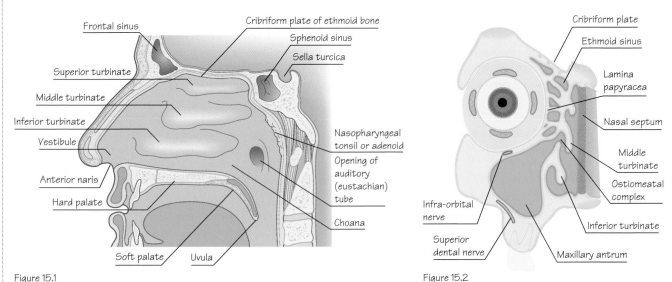

Figure 15.1
The lateral nasal wall

Figure 15.2
The paranasal sinuses

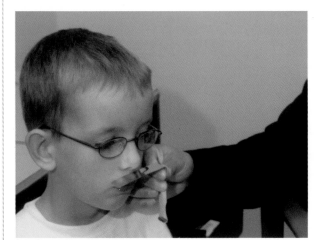

Figure 15.3
The mist test
Testing the nasal airway

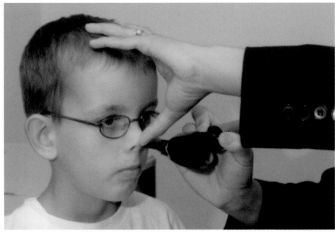

Figure 15.4
Auriscope
An auriscope can be used to examine the nose if you do not have access to an endoscope

The nasal cavities extend from the vestibule in front to the nasopharynx behind. The nasal septum (made of cartilage and bone) separates the nose into two nasal cavities. The soft cartilaginous septum can be distorted during birth or in later life as a result of injury. A deviated nasal septum is common and can sometimes cause a blocked nose and can be treated surgically if required (see Chapter 17).

The rich blood supply to the nasal cavities is derived from both the internal and external carotid artery systems (see Chapter 16). Venous drainage is through valveless veins that follow the arterial pattern and have direct communication with the cavernous sinuses. This has a bearing on spread of infection to the intracranial cavity.

The nasal vestibule is lined with squamous epithelium. The nasal cavity itself is covered with pseudo-stratified ciliated columnar respiratory epithelium, rich in seromucinous glands. Figure 15.1 outlines the anatomy of the lateral nasal wall, where the paranasal sinuses and the lacrimal duct drain.

Paranasal sinuses

The paranasal sinuses are a network of air-filled spaces lined with respiratory mucosa (pseudo-stratified columnar squamous epithelium). They extend from the nasal cavities and occupy part of the skeleton of the mid-face and the skull (Figure 15.2). The mucosa is rich with mucous-producing goblet cells. Infection or inflammation in the nose can occur in these sinuses resulting in sinusitis (see Chapters 19 and 20).

There are maxillary (paired), frontal and sphenoid sinuses. Additionally, there are multiple, small, air-filled spaces on each side collectively referred to as the ethmoid sinus complexes. The maxillary sinuses are present at birth and are the largest pair of sinuses, each consisting of a large cavity referred to as the maxillary antrum (Figure 15.2). The ethmoid sinuses are very close to the orbit and the brain and these also have very thin walls, hence sinus infection can spread to cause severe orbital infections, brain abscess and meningitis. They are separated from the orbit by a thin plate of bone referred to as the lamina papyracea (Figure 15.2).

The internal carotid artery, optic nerve and cavernous sinus are very closely related to the sphenoid sinuses and can be affected by disease processes in this area, as well as being at risk during sphenoid sinus surgery.

Physiology

The nose is designed not only to act as a conduit for air entering the respiratory tract, but to warm and moisten air as it passes through (humidification). The bony projections from the lateral nasal wall (turbinates) are lined with mucosa and help with this process (Figure 15.1). Currents are generated by inspired air coming in contact with this mucosa. The turbinates and the nasal mucosa in general can change size rapidly due to rapid alterations in blood flow called the nasal cycle. The ciliated respiratory mucosa also filters particulate matter from inspired air.

The olfactory mucosa is a small strip of specialised neuro-epithelium that responds to chemicals and transmits the sense of smell to the brain.

The function of paranasal sinuses is not fully understood. Some possible roles that have been postulated include reducing skull weight by having air-filled spaces in the bony facial skeleton, to aid air humidification and warming, playing a part in sound resonance (disease processes can alter voice quality) and increasing the surface area for olfactory mucosa.

Examination of the nose

A good way to test the nasal airway is to put a cold spatula under the nostrils and look for condensation – the mist test (Figure 15.3). This is especially useful in children. Remember that the state of engorgement of the nasal mucosa fluctuates between each nostril and between day and night.

Always examine the nose in a good light, preferably using a headlight or a good quality torch. If these are not available, an auriscope can be gently inserted into the nostril to look at the nose – ask the patient to breathe through their mouth or the auriscope lens will mist up (Figure 15.4). Check if the septum is midline, look at the turbinates, look for mucopus and check for polyps and swellings. An ENT surgeon will be able to carry out a more thorough examination using a rigid endoscope (see Figures 20.2 and 20.3), but you can get a good preliminary idea about nasal pathology using very simple instruments looking backwards, not upwards.

Clinical practice point

Remember that the nose runs backwards, not upwards, so look along the plane of the hard palate, not upwards to the patient's eyes.

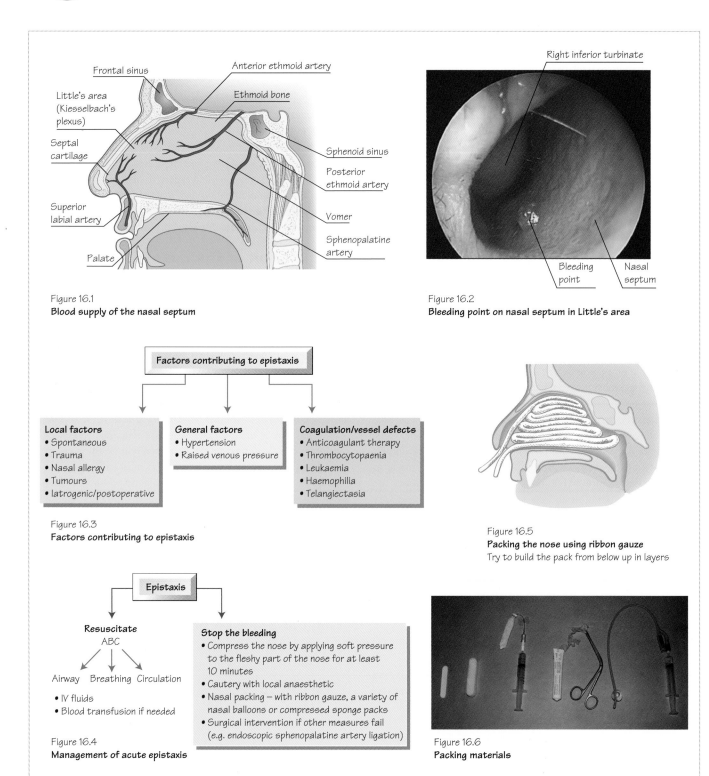

Figure 16.1
Blood supply of the nasal septum

Labels: Frontal sinus, Little's area (Kiesselbach's plexus), Septal cartilage, Superior labial artery, Palate, Anterior ethmoid artery, Ethmoid bone, Sphenoid sinus, Posterior ethmoid artery, Vomer, Sphenopalatine artery

Figure 16.2
Bleeding point on nasal septum in Little's area

Labels: Right inferior turbinate, Bleeding point, Nasal septum

Factors contributing to epistaxis

Local factors
- Spontaneous
- Trauma
- Nasal allergy
- Tumours
- Iatrogenic/postoperative

General factors
- Hypertension
- Raised venous pressure

Coagulation/vessel defects
- Anticoagulant therapy
- Thrombocytopaenia
- Leukaemia
- Haemophilia
- Telangiectasia

Figure 16.3
Factors contributing to epistaxis

Figure 16.5
Packing the nose using ribbon gauze
Try to build the pack from below up in layers

Epistaxis

Resuscitate
ABC

Airway   Breathing   Circulation

- IV fluids
- Blood transfusion if needed

Stop the bleeding
- Compress the nose by applying soft pressure to the fleshy part of the nose for at least 10 minutes
- Cautery with local anaesthetic
- Nasal packing – with ribbon gauze, a variety of nasal balloons or compressed sponge packs
- Surgical intervention if other measures fail (e.g. endoscopic sphenopalatine artery ligation)

Figure 16.4
Management of acute epistaxis

Figure 16.6
Packing materials

Ear, Nose and Throat at a Glance, First Edition. Nazia Munir and Ray Clarke.

38 © 2013 Nazia Munir and Ray Clarke. Published 2013 by Blackwell Publishing Ltd.

Applied basic science

Nosebleeds (epistaxis) are common. They occur mainly in children and in middle-aged and elderly adults. A nosebleed can be fatal. The nose has a rich blood supply (Figure 16.1). A network of vessels derived from both the internal and external carotid arteries converge in the nasal septum in Little's area or Kiesselbach's plexus. This is a common site of bleeding (Figure 16.2).

Air flows over this area during respiration. It can become dried with crusted secretions and a vessel wall can break through the mucosa causing a bleed. Children often have a prominent vein running just above the junction between the skin and the mucosa of the nasal septum known as a retrocolumellar vein. This area is also prone to bleeding.

Usually, a nosebleed settles quickly as the vessels contract and a clot develops. In elderly patients with cardiovascular disease (atheroma) the vessel can stay open and the bleeding is prolonged. Nosebleeds can be spontaneous or can be brought about by a very mild trauma to the nose including digital trauma or nose picking.

Aetiology

Most nosebleeds are idiopathic (i.e. they occur spontaneously without any definite cause). Some of the factors that can make a nose bleed more likely are shown in Figure 16.3.

Management of epistaxis

There are two aspects to the treatment of nosebleeds: management of the acute bleed and treatment of recurrent epistaxis – usually in children.

1 *The acute bleed* The two aims of treatment are to resuscitate the patient and to stem the bleeding (Figure 16.4). Nasal packing (Figures 16.5 and 16.6) or surgical intervention may be required to stop the bleeding.

2 *Management of recurrent nosebleeds*
- May only need reassurance and no treatment if mild and has stopped
- Treat the underlying condition (e.g. nasal allergy)
- Use a cream or ointment (e.g. Naseptin cream® applied twice daily to Little's area)
- Severe cases may need nasal cautery in the ENT clinic under local anaesthetic using, for example, silver nitrate.

Complications

A nosebleed is at the very least a nuisance. In children, clothes may be stained and the child sent home from school. This can be very troublesome if the bleeds are recurrent. A massive bleed can, if prolonged, cause exsanguination and shock, usually in an adult.

Clinical practice point

Recurrent nosebleeds in children are common and, unless there are unusual clinical factors, there is no need for invasive investigations. A prolonged bleed in an adult will require hospital admission.

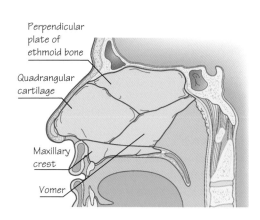

Perpendicular plate of ethmoid bone

Quadrangular cartilage

Maxillary crest

Vomer

Figure 17.1
The nasal septum

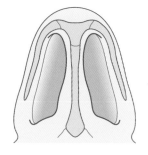

Figure 17.2a
Straight nasal septum

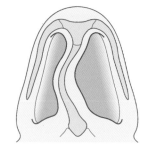

Figure 17.2b
Deviated nasal septum

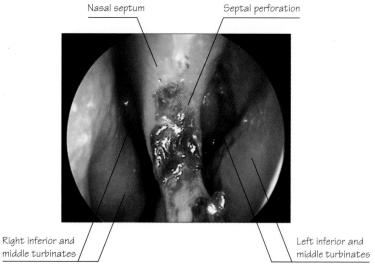

Nasal septum

Septal perforation

Right inferior and middle turbinates

Left inferior and middle turbinates

Figure 17.3
Nasal septal perforation
Note small amount of crusting over the edge of the perforation. Also note that both right and left nasal passages are visible simultaneously through the septal perforation

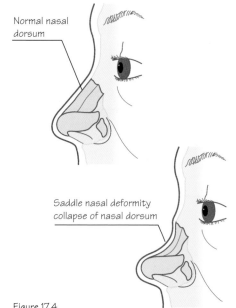

Normal nasal dorsum

Saddle nasal deformity collapse of nasal dorsum

Figure 17.4
'Saddle nose'
Saddling is often the result of late treatment of a traumatic septal haematoma causing damage to the supporting cartilaginous structure of the nose

Ear, Nose and Throat at a Glance, First Edition. Nazia Munir and Ray Clarke.

The nasal septum is composed of cartilaginous and bony components (Figure 17.1). It is covered with mucoperichondrium and mucoperiosteum, from which it derives its blood supply. It divides the nasal cavity into two. The septum provides some of the support of external nose and contributes to nasal shape.

Septal deviation

The septum is often slightly deviated to one side or other. This usually causes no trouble but a more severely angulated or dislocated nasal septum will cause one or both nasal passages to partly obstruct (Figure 17.2). The patient complains of a blocked nose and drainage of the sinuses can be affected. They may also complain about the shape of the nose and of reduced sense of smell (hyposmia), or no smell (anosmia). In many cases no treatment is needed; more severe cases may warrant surgical correction – a septoplasty.

Septal perforation

A perforated nasal septum (Figure 17.3) can be completely asymptomatic. If there is crusting and debris around the edges, the patient may complain of nosebleeds. Some patients complain of whistling noises as air goes across the perforation. Surgical correction of septal perforation is not easy. Symptoms can be helped by getting the patient to use glycerine or saline drops to moisten the nose or by inserting a prosthesis (septal button) to occlude the perforation.

Causes of septal perforation

- Trauma
- Surgery
- Infections (e.g. syphilis, tuberculosis)
- Vasculitic conditions (e.g. Wegener's granulomatosis)
- Recreational drug use (e.g. cocaine)

Septal haematoma

Nasal injury can result in the formation of a septal haematoma (see Chapter 18). This is a bleed under the perichondrium lining the septal cartilage. The cartilage derives its blood supply from the overlying mucosa and this is disrupted by formation of a haematoma. Cartilage necrosis may occur if this is not treated quickly with drainage of the haematoma. As a consequence a septal perforation may occur. If the parts of the cartilaginous septum crucial in providing support to the nasal dorsum are destroyed, a saddle deformity of the nose occurs (Figure 17.4).

Alar collapse

Not strictly speaking a septal pathology, alar collapse occurs when the skin and cartilage of the lateral nasal wall prolapse inwards on inspiration, especially sniffing. It is fairly common in elderly patients as the tissues become less elastic in old age.

Clinical practice points

- Most nasal septal deviations are asymptomatic and do not require intervention.
- Septal haematomas need to be specifically looked for in cases of nasal trauma.

ENT trauma I

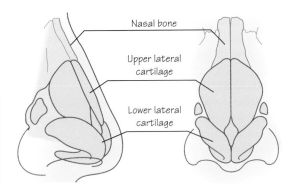

Nasal bone

Upper lateral
cartilage

Lower lateral
cartilage

Figure 18.1
Skeletal structure of the nose

Fractured
nasal bones

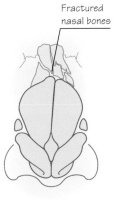

Figure 18.2
Fractured nasal bones

Septal
haematoma

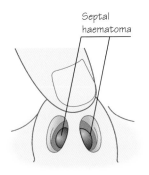

Figure 18.3
Bilateral septal haematoma

ENT trauma II

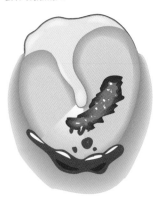

Figure 18.4
**Traumatic perforation of the
left eardrum**

Vertebral
column

Anterior
commisure

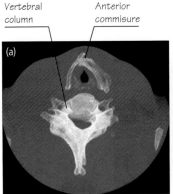
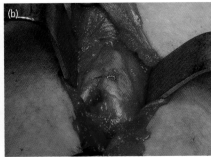

Figure 18.5
(a) CT Scan of laryngeal fracture
(b) The fracture has been stabilised by anchoring the two laminas of the thyroid cartilage

All head and neck trauma cases should initially be evaluated and managed as closed head injuries. The head and neck has a very rich blood supply and consequently brisk bleeding is often present but this should not distract from prompt, systematic evaluation of the patient. Swift assessment of the airway, breathing, circulation and cervical spine is imperative. A thorough systematic secondary survey is also essential.

Nasal trauma

The nose is particularly prone to injury as a result of its prominent central location and the low tensile strength of its skeleton (Figure 18.1). A combination of soft tissue injury, nasal bone fracture, septal deviation/fracture/haematoma or cerebrospinal fluid (CSF) leak may occur. Typical symptoms of nasal injury include:
- Epistaxis (nose bleed)
- Noticeable cosmetic deformity
- Nasal airway compromise.

Peri-orbital and subconjunctival bruising (ecchymosis) may also be present. Nasal trauma often occurs in conjunction with other maxillofacial injuries and these need to be carefully excluded.

It is important to note the nature of the injury and any previous history of trauma or nasal deformity. The nasal septum should be assessed for any obvious deformity or a septal haematoma. Unless seen almost immediately after the trauma, soft tissue swelling and tenderness makes clinical assessment challenging. In uncomplicated cases, it is advisable to reassess the patient in 5–7 days following the injury, allowing time for the bruising and swelling to subside. Radiological investigations have no role in uncomplicated nasal injuries, but may be useful in the presence of other maxillofacial injuries.

Management is dependent on the nature and extent of injury.

Soft tissue injuries

Wounds should be débrided and cleaned. Abrasions are best left open to heal and simple steristrips may be used to close small lacerations. Larger wounds should be sutured. Tetanus immunisation status needs to be ascertained and cover ensured in the presence of an open wound.

Epistaxis

Epistaxis is common with nasal injuries. Most cases resolve with conservative measures and application of direct pressure. If there is a nasal fracture, closed fracture reduction may be needed to stop the bleeding. In persistent cases nasal packing may be needed to arrest the bleeding.

Nasal bone fracture

Uncomplicated fractures without a cosmetic or functional problem only require simple reassurance and no intervention. With simple displaced fractures (Figure 18.2) closed reduction under local or general anaesthetic may be required. Fracture reduction should be carried out either immediately after the injury (before marked soft tissue swelling sets in) or 5–7 days after the injury (to allow distortion due to swelling to resolve).

After 2 weeks the fractured bones start to fix. Fracture reduction after this period can be very difficult if not impossible. Such delays should therefore be avoided. Open fractures may necessitate general anaesthesia and open reduction. If there is malunion of nasal bones a formal septorhinoplasty procedure may be needed.

Septal haematoma

Haematoma (unilateral or bilateral) formation under the perichondrium separates the perichondrium from the septal cartilage (Figure 18.3). Septal cartilage relies on the perichondrium for blood supply. If the haematoma is left untreated for more than 48 hours cartilage necrosis occurs.

Septal haematoma usually presents with progressive nasal obstruction. A large, soft, bluish–red swelling is seen on examination and may be confused with nasal polyps, septal deviation or enlarged turbinates.

Treatment is prompt and adequate drainage. Needle aspiration may suffice before a clot has formed, otherwise a formal incision and drainage is necessary. If not treated promptly a septal abscess and cartilage necrosis result, causing a saddle nose deformity and functional deficit (see Chapter 17).

CSF leak

Cerebrospinal fluid (CSF) leak should be suspected if there is clear nasal discharge (rhinorrhoea) following nasal injury. The cribriform plate is extremely thin and can be damaged in nasal injuries.

The clear discharge should be tested for glucose content (similar to serum levels) and 2 transferrin (protein present in perilymph and CSF). Most CSF leaks resolve spontaneously. Persistent leaks may need surgical repair.

The patient is at risk of developing meningitis until the leak stops and he/she should be made aware of this risk. The role of prophylactic antibiotics is controversial.

ENT trauma: II

Ear trauma

The external, middle or inner ear may be involved in traumatic injury.

Auricular haematoma

The auricle or pinna is readily accessible to trauma because of its location. Shearing forces from blunt injuries disrupt the adherence of auricular perichondrium from the underlying cartilage, resulting in the formation of a subperichondrial haematoma. This deprives the cartilage (which lacks an intrinsic blood supply) of nutrition. If an auricular haematoma is left untreated infection, fibrosis and cartilage necrosis occur, resulting in auricular deformity ('cauliflower ear').

Treatment consists of drainage of the haematoma and application of a pressure dressing to allow re-apposition of the perichondrium to the cartilage, preventing cartilage necrosis and auricular deformity (see Chapter 5).

Tympanic membrane perforation

The most common cause of tympanic membrane perforation is infection. However, blunt trauma, barotrauma or direct injury (e.g. with a cotton bud inserted in the ear) can also result in tympanic membrane perforation (Figure 18.4). The patient may be asymptomatic or may complain of hearing loss, bloody or serous otorrhoea, or ear discomfort aggravated by wind or cold weather. Most traumatic perforations heal spontaneously within 6 weeks. The ear should be kept dry until the perforation has healed. In cases where the perforation does not heal spontaneously, surgical reconstruction (myringoplasty) may be considered if the patient is symptomatic.

Haemotympanum

Blunt trauma to the middle ear can cause a bleed behind an intact eardrum (haemotympanum). This causes a conductive deafness – usually temporary – and is typically short-lived, resolving without the need for intervention.

Ossicular injury

Head trauma can result in displacement or discontinuity of the ossicles resulting in a conductive hearing loss. Displacement of the stapes can result in sensorineural hearing loss.

There is frequently an associated haemotympanum. If the hearing loss persists after the haemotympanum has resolved the patient should be referred for a specialist opinion to consider options for hearing reconstruction and rehabilitation.

Temporal bone fractures

The temporal bone is a very complex anatomical structure and forms part of the base of skull. It contains the hearing and balance organs as well as the facial nerve, carotid artery and jugular vein.

Fractures of the temporal bone most commonly result from high impact blunt trauma and can extend along the whole of the skull base. Symptoms and signs related to temporal bone fractures include hearing loss (conductive, sensorineural, or mixed), vertigo (dizziness), otalgia, bloody and/or CSF otorrhoea/rhinorrhoea, tympanic membrane perforation and haemotympanum. The Battle sign (ecchymosis of the post-auricular skin) and the 'raccoon sign' (ecchymosis of the periorbital area) may also be present. The fracture may also involve the temporomandibular (jaw) joint.

Patients with temporal bone fractures often have multiple injuries and initial assessment and management of the patient should be according to the Advance Trauma Life Support (ATLS) guidelines. There may be associated maxillofacial and intracranial injuries as well as potential trauma to other regions. The cervical spine should be stabilised, assessed and cleared of injury before the head is manipulated.

The clinical examination should include a full neuro-otological examination, as well as a complete nose and throat examination. Once the patient's condition has been stabilised and any life or limb-threatening emergencies dealt with, tuning fork tests and pure tone audiometry should be performed to obtain a baseline hearing assessment. For uncomplicated temporal bone trauma a computed tomography (CT) scan of the head will exclude intracranial injury and identify any fractures. A high resolution CT scan of the temporal bones is required in complicated cases such as those with facial paralysis, CSF leak or vascular injury. Early specialist input is required for these cases.

Neck trauma

Neck trauma is increasingly common due to gunshot injuries, stabbings and road traffic accidents. All head and neck injuries should initially be managed as closed head injuries as above with appropriate evaluation of airway, breathing, circulation and cervical spine.

Severe neck injuries may necessitate endotracheal intubation or, in extreme cases, a tracheostomy. A penetrating wound to the neck can cause an injury to the neurovascular structures, laryngotracheal or pharyngo-oesophageal structures. It nearly always warrants surgical exploration.

Laryngeal injury

The larynx comprises a complex arrangement of cartilage, nerves and muscles covered by a mucous membrane lining. Laryngeal structures can become dislocated or fractured in trauma. Traumatic laryngeal injuries are fortunately very rare but can result in serious life-threatening airway compromise (Figure 18.5). Therefore, such injuries should be recognised early and treated promptly.

Very severe injuries are usually clearly evident and frequently fatal. Patients with less severe injuries may present with acute onset of hoarseness/change in voice, haemoptysis, dysphagia, odynophagia, anterior neck pain, dyspnoea, stridor, surgical emphysema or soft tissue swelling/ecchymosis on the anterior neck.

Management should be as per ATLS guidelines, with airway protection and maintenance being the paramount immediate concern. Cervical spine injury should also be suspected and excluded in such cases. These patients should be dealt with by a team adept at providing initial acute airway management and specialist input should be sought early.

Clinical practice points

• All head and neck trauma patients should initially be evaluated and managed as closed head injuries. Management should be as per ATLS guidelines.
• Uncomplicated nasal fractures without a cosmetic or functional problem only require simple reassurance and no intervention.
• Laryngeal trauma is very rare, but can be fatal and specialist input should be sought early.

19 Acute rhinosinusitis

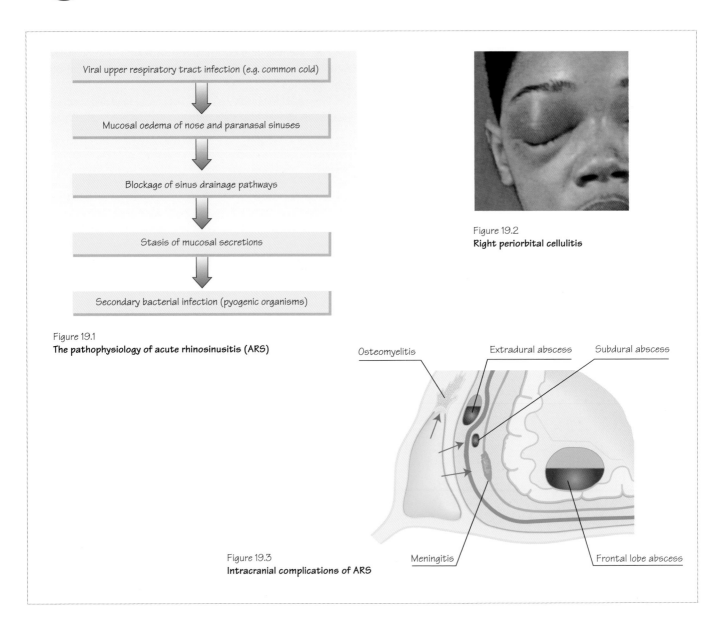

Viral upper respiratory tract infection (e.g. common cold)

⬇

Mucosal oedema of nose and paranasal sinuses

⬇

Blockage of sinus drainage pathways

⬇

Stasis of mucosal secretions

⬇

Secondary bacterial infection (pyogenic organisms)

Figure 19.1
The pathophysiology of acute rhinosinusitis (ARS)

Figure 19.2
Right periorbital cellulitis

Osteomyelitis Extradural abscess Subdural abscess

Meningitis Frontal lobe abscess

Figure 19.3
Intracranial complications of ARS

Definition
Acute rhinosinusitis (ARS) is an acute inflammatory condition of the nose and paranasal sinuses. As the mucosal lining of the nose and paranasal sinuses are continuous, ARS is a more appropriate term than the traditionally used acute sinusitis.

ARS is defined as (European Position Paper on Rhinosinusitis and Nasal Polyps – EPOS 2007):
• Sudden onset of two or more symptoms, one of which should be either nasal blockage/obstruction/congestion or nasal discharge (anterior/posterior nasal drip)

  ± Facial pain/pressure

  ± Loss/reduction of sense of smell

• Symptoms lasting less than 12 weeks
• In recurrent ARS, there must be symptom-free intervals present.

Pathophysiology
ARS usually develops as a result of a preceding viral upper respiratory tract infection which leads secondarily to a bacterial infection (Figure 19.1). Most of the sinuses drain in the middle meatus and congestion and obstruction of this part of the sino-nasal anatomy is often implicated in ARS.

Cilia beat to guide secretions towards the natural sinus ostia for drainage. Blockage of the sinuses as a result of inflammation

Ear, Nose and Throat at a Glance, First Edition. Nazia Munir and Ray Clarke.

prevents drainage and results in stasis of mucous secretions, leading to development of an environment in which bacterial infection flourishes.

The most commonly implicated bacterial pathogens are the pyogenic or pus-forming organisms such as *Streptococcus pneumoniae*, *Haemophilus influenzae* and *Moraxella catarrhalis*.

Presence of atopy, anatomical abnormalities (such as septal deviation and mechanical obstruction to sinus drainage pathways) and a history of chronic rhinosinusitis (with or without nasal polyposis) may predispose some individuals to developing ARS. Sinonasal tumours and foreign bodies can also cause mechanical obstruction. Conditions affecting mucociliary clearance (e.g. cystic fibrosis, Kartagener's syndrome) as well as immunodeficiency disorders are also risk factors for recurrent ARS.

Clinical features

The diagnosis of ARS is predominantly based on clinical history and examination. Patients usually present with a history of a preceding coryzal illness with clear rhinorrhoea, nasal congestion, fever and malaise, followed by development of symptoms of ARS:

• Prurulent rhinorrhoea
• Nasal congestion (more marked)
• Facial pain and/or pressure
• Hyposmia or altered taste
• Dental pain.

On examination, there is often mucopus in one or both nasal cavities. Gentle palpation of the surface of the involved sinus can be painful. The patient may complain of a severe headache, particularly over the frontal region.

There is no role for plain X-rays or aspiration of sinus contents. These procedures are rarely performed for confirmation of diagnosis unless in specialist ENT care.

Management

Treatment is aimed at symptom control and prevention of disease progression and complications. Most cases of ARS can be managed in the primary care setting with good analgesia, decongestants and appropriate antibiotics. However, a high index of suspicion needs to be maintained in resistant or non-responsive cases for development of complications – in such scenarios an early specialist ENT opinion is advisable. Broadly speaking, the treatment of ARS includes:
• Analgesics (paracetamol ± non-steroidal anti-inflammatory drugs)
• Decongestants (topical and/or systemic)
• Antibiotics (e.g. amoxicillin, cephalosporins)
• Rarely, surgical intervention.

Complications

Most cases of ARS resolve without adverse effects. The anatomical location of the nose and paranasal sinuses, however, means that the infection can spread to adjacent areas.

The most frequent complication of ARS, most notably in children, is development of periorbital cellulitis (Figure 19.2). Infection can spread directly through the thin bone separating the sinuses from the orbit (lamina papyracea) or by venous thrombophlebitis. If not treated promptly, this can rapidly progress to orbital cellulitis, subperiosteal and/or orbital abscess formation, blindness and cavernous sinus thrombosis, which can be fatal.

An urgent specialist review and, in most cases, hospital admission for intravenous antibiotics and monitoring of visual acuity is required if any degree of orbital involvement is suspected. As inpatients, these cases are managed in a multidisciplinary manner with involvement from ENT surgeons, ophthalmologists and paediatricians in the case of children. Radiological imaging (CT scanning) is utilised in patients who have severe symptoms at the outset or in those whose symptoms continue to progress or do not respond to maximal medical therapy. Surgical intervention is required if there is evidence of abscess formation.

Osteomyelitis, meningitis, extradural/subdural and intracranial abscesses can also be sequelae of ARS (Figure 19.3). Osteomyelitis of the frontal bone can result in the formation of a subperiosteal abscess on the forehead and is referred to as 'Pott's puffy tumour'. Subdural abscess is the most common intracranial complication. It may occur via direct extension through the posterior wall of the frontal sinus or infection may spread through thrombophlebitis of the valveless veins (see Chapter 15). A high index of suspicion needs to be maintained in cases with severe headaches, swinging pyrexia and any neurological symptoms and signs. Urgent ENT or neurological opinion should be sought in these cases. Delayed diagnosis can result in long-term neurological deficits and even fatality.

A long-standing untreated sinus infection can cause persistent chronic obstruction to the drainage pathway of the sinus so that the bone expands and causes an external deformity – known as a mucocele. These can progressively expand concentrically and result in bony erosion and extension beyond the sinus and should be referred for early specialist input and management.

Multiple repeated episodes of acute sinusitis can cause severe inflammation of the nasal mucosa and can sometimes develop into chronic rhinosinusitis.

Clinical practice points

• ARS is very common and most cases resolve without any long-term sequelae.
• However, a high index of suspicion for complications of ARS should be maintained and referral for specialist opinion should be made early if in any doubt.

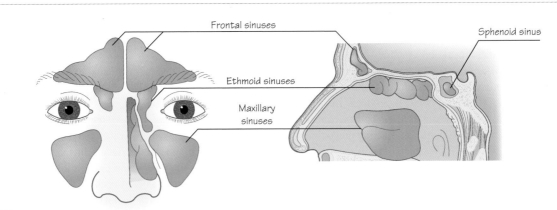

Figure 20.1
The paranasal sinuses
All of these can be accessed endo-nasally using rigid nasoendoscopes (see Figure 20.2)

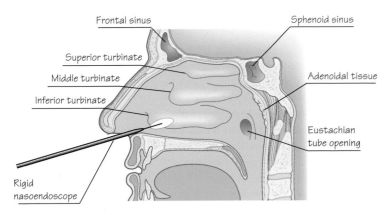

Figure 20.2
Rigid nasoendoscopy
This is a valuable diagnostic tool as well as being essential for performing endonasal surgical procedures such as functional endoscopic sinus surgery (FESS). Endoscopes with lenses at a variety of angles (0, 30, 45 and 70 degree) are available to get a better view around corners and difficult to access areas

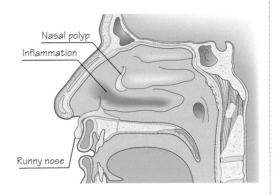

Figure 20.3
Lateral nasal wall with some features of chronic rhinosinusitis (CRS)

Definitions

Rhinosinusitis is one of the more prevalent chronic illnesses worldwide, affecting individuals of all ages. It is an inflammatory process that involves the nose and paranasal sinuses. Rhinosinusitis may be acute (ARS) or chronic (CRS). CRS can be subject to acute exacerbations. CRS can cause a significant degree of morbidity and it can reduce the individual's quality of life and their productivity.

Rhinosinusitis is defined as (European Position Paper on Rhinosinusitis and Nasal Polyps – EPOS 2007):
• Inflammation of the nose and paranasal sinuses characterised by two or more of the following symptoms, one of which must be nasal blockage, obstruction, congestion or nasal discharge:

± facial pain or pressure
± reduction or loss of smell
and either
• Endoscopic signs of:
  • polyps, and/or
  • mucopurulent discharge primarily from middle meatus, and/or
  • oedema and/or mucosal obstruction primarily in middle meatus
  and/or
• Computed tomography (CT) changes:
  • mucosal changes within the osteomeatal complex or sinuses.

It is termed CRS if the symptoms last for more than 12 weeks without complete resolution.

Ear, Nose and Throat at a Glance, First Edition. Nazia Munir and Ray Clarke.

Pathophysiology

CRS is predominantly a multifactorial inflammatory disease. There are four pairs of paranasal sinuses lined with ciliated, pseudo-stratified, columnar epithelium (Figure 20.1). Goblet cells are interspersed among the columnar cells. The mucosa is attached directly to the bone. The maxillary, frontal and anterior ethmoid sinuses drain through their ostia located at the osteo-meatal complex lying lateral to the middle turbinate (middle meatus) and the posterior ethmoid and sphenoid sinuses open behind the superior turbinate (superior meatus; Figure 20.2).

Mechanical obstruction of the drainage pathways, increased mucus production (e.g. with an upper respiratory tract infection) and impaired ciliary function (e.g. cystic fibrosis) lead to stasis of secretions within the sinuses and resultant inflammation. Stasis of secretion results in cessation of bacterial export, propagating mucosal inflammation and compromising aeration of the mucosa. This in turn leads to increased ciliary dysfunction and the vicious cycle continues, resulting in CRS.

Other aetiological factors contributing to CRS include the following:
• Allergy and atopy
• Other airway disease (e.g. asthma)
• Fungi inducing an eosinophilic reaction (e.g. *Aspergillus* spp.)
• Bacterial super-antigens
• Persistent low grade infection (biofilms, osteitis)
• Non-steroidal anti-inflammatory drug sensitivity
• Ciliary dysfunction (e.g. cystic fibrosis, Kartagener's syndrome)
• Immune dysfunction
• Genetic predisposition
• Environmental factors.

Nasal polyps

CRS may occur with or without nasal polyps. Nasal polyps are oedematous overgrowths of the nasal and paranasal sinus mucosa (Figure 20.3). They are mostly covered with pseudo-stratified epithelium with ciliated cells and goblet cells and are comprised of loose connective tissue, oedema, inflammatory cells, some glands and capillaries. The most common inflammatory cells present in nasal polyps are eosinophils; interleukin 5 is the predominant cytokine.

It is not known why some individuals with CRS are more likely to develop nasal polyps. However, there is a notably higher incidence of nasal polyps in individuals with asthma and sensitivity to non-steroidal anti-inflammatory drugs (this is referred to as Samster's triad).

Clinical features

A thorough and concise history of symptoms and potential exacerbating and risk factors is mandatory. In contrast to acute rhinosinusitis (see Chapter 19), the signs and symptoms of CRS can be much more subtle. CRS patients can present with a range of symptoms including the following:
• Nasal congestion or stuffiness
• Rhinorrhoea or nasal discharge
• Post-nasal drip

• Facial pain or pressure
• Change or loss in sense of smell
• Altered taste
• Dry or sore throat
• Halitosis
• Worsening of asthma
• Sneezing
• Itchy or runny eyes
• Blocked ears
• General malaise.

Clinical examination

Clinical examination should include a full head and neck examination. A complete nasal examination should include direct visualisation of the nasal cavities using a rigid nasoendoscope (Figure 20.2). Endoscopic findings may show one or more of the following:
• Nasal mucosal inflammation
• Nasal polyps
• Mucopurulent secretions
• Turbinate hypertrophy
• Other anatomic abnormalities (e.g. nasal septal deviation causing obstruction).

Management

The mainstay of CRS management is medical therapy using a combination of topical and oral steroids, antibiotics and saline nasal irrigation. The aim of medical treatment is to reduce mucosal inflammation and polyposis, promote sinus drainage and eradicate any underlying low-grade infection. Most patients with CRS respond well to medical therapy and do not require any further intervention.

If there is a history suggestive of underlying allergic aetiology, testing such as skin prick tests can help identify allergens and the patient can accordingly be given advice on allergen avoidance. Anti-histamines are also be useful and can be given topically or systemically.

Surgical intervention acts as an adjunct to medical treatment and is used in cases that have not responded adequately to medical therapy. Surgery is performed using rigid endoscopes (Figure 20.2) and is referred to as functional endoscopic sinus surgery (FESS). The goal of surgery is to re-establish anatomical sinus drainage pathways and ventilation, aiming to restore the functional integrity of the inflamed mucosal lining. A significant proportion of patients will require continued medical therapy after FESS.

Clinical practice points

• CRS can cause a significant degree of morbidity, and it can reduce the individual's quality of life and their productivity.
• The mainstay of CRS management is medical therapy.
• Surgical intervention acts as an adjunct to medical treatment.

The pharynx and oesophagus: basic science and examination

21

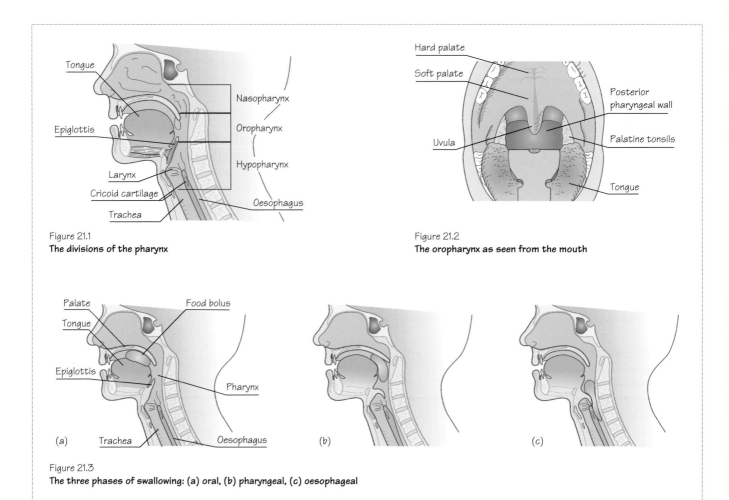

Figure 21.1
The divisions of the pharynx

Figure 21.2
The oropharynx as seen from the mouth

Figure 21.3
The three phases of swallowing: (a) oral, (b) pharyngeal, (c) oesophageal

Ear, Nose and Throat at a Glance, First Edition. Nazia Munir and Ray Clarke.
© 2013 Nazia Munir and Ray Clarke. Published 2013 by Blackwell Publishing Ltd.

The pharynx

The pharynx is the upper part of the combined air and food passages (aero-digestive tract). It leads to the oesophagus and is divided for descriptive purposes into three parts (Figure 21.1): the nasopharynx, the oropharynx (Figure 21.2) and the hypopharynx. The nasopharynx is between the skull base and the level of the hard palate and contains the adenoids (in children) and the entrance to the Eustachian tubes. The boundaries of the oropharynx are the level of the hard palate down to the level of the vallecula – this is the junction between the base of the tongue and the epiglottis. The structures within the oropharynx include the tonsils, base of the tongue and the soft palate. The hypopharynx extends between the level of the vallecula to the cricopharynx which is the muscular sphincter at the upper end of the oesophagus.

Swallowing

The main function of the pharynx as related to the digestive tract is to ensure that chewed and partly digested food is propelled from the mouth into the oesophagus. The process of swallowing takes place in three phases (Figure 21.3):

1 The oral phase commences by chewing which starts the digestion process by breaking down large food pieces. This along with saliva secretion from the major and minor salivary glands moistens the food which is then passed along the back of the tongue into the oropharynx. The tongue is an integral part of the oral phase of swallowing to allow the food bolus to be formed and propelled backwards into the oropharynx by the base of the tongue.

2 In the pharyngeal phase the muscles around the larynx close and push the food bolus into the oesophagus. These muscles are known as the pharyngeal constrictors. During this phase the larynx elevates to protect the airway and lower respiratory tract.

3 In the oesophageal phase of swallowing the food passes through the oesophagus and into the stomach.

Aspiration

It is important that no food or fluid passes from the pharynx into the trachea and lungs during swallowing. The movements of the pharyngeal and laryngeal muscles protect the airway. If this mechanism fails the patient may aspirate which can cause serious respiratory problems.

Examination of the pharynx

The nasopharynx and the hypopharynx are difficult to examine without the use of a flexible fibreoptic endoscope or a mirror placed in the back of the mouth. However, the oropharynx can be easily visualised using a good light source and tongue depressor (Figure 21.2). The oral cavity is examined at the same time as part of a full ENT and head and neck examination.

Clinical practice point

Swallowing is a complex process requiring coordination of the muscles of the oral cavity, pharynx and larynx. Loss of function of any of these stages can cause potential aspiration and a lower respiratory tract infection.

---

22 The nasopharynx and adenoids

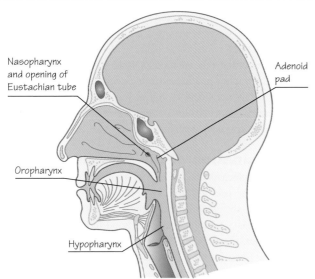

Nasopharynx and opening of Eustachian tube

Adenoid pad

Oropharynx

Hypopharynx

Figure 22.1
Anatomy of the pharynx

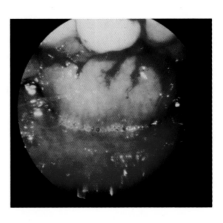

Figure 22.2
Endoscopic view of the adenoids

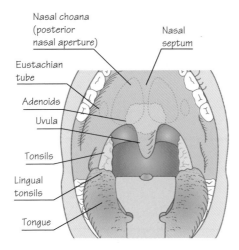

Nasal choana (posterior nasal aperture)

Nasal septum

Eustachian tube

Adenoids

Uvula

Tonsils

Lingual tonsils

Tongue

Figure 22.3
The adenoids
The adenoids are not usually seen as they are behind the soft palate

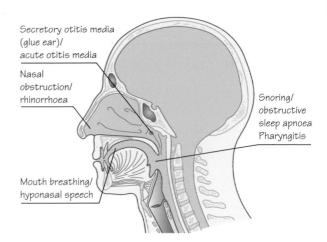

Secretory otitis media (glue ear)/ acute otitis media

Nasal obstruction/ rhinorrhoea

Snoring/ obstructive sleep apnoea
Pharyngitis

Mouth breathing/ hyponasal speech

Figure 22.4
Clinical features of adenoid hypertrophy

The nasopharynx

The upper part of the pharynx above and behind the hard palate is referred to as the nasopharynx. It lies close to the skull base and the posterior openings (choanae) of the nose. It contains the adenoids and the openings of the Eustachian tubes (Figure 22.1).

Adenoids

Adenoids are a collection of lymphoid tissue (Figures 22.2 and 22.3). They are part of a circle of lymphoid tissue known as Waldeyer's ring that surrounds the entrance to the pharynx and respiratory tract. The other parts of the ring include the lingual tonsils on the base of the tongue and the pharyngeal tonsils.

Adenoids are very small at birth, reach maximum size at the age of about 5–7 years, and then regress. Adults have little or no adenoid tissue. They have the same function as lymphoid tissue elsewhere (i.e. to mount an immunological response to infection).

In some children repeated infections cause the adenoids to enlarge and obstruct the airway. Figure 22.4 illustrates the symptoms that can arise as a result of adenoid hypertrophy. They can contribute to sleep disordered breathing and obstructive sleep apnoea (see Chapter 27). Adenoids are also implicated in the aetiology of middle ear effusions (also known as otitis media with effusion, OME, or glue ear) and acute otitis media. Gross enlargement of the adenoids obstructing the Eustachian tubes causes pressure change in the middle ear which can result in OME. If this occurs with spread of infection to the middle ear along the Eustachian tube, then an acute middle ear infection arises. Obstruction of the nasopharynx also results in persistent mouth breathing and hyponasal speech in children.

As adenoids are an aggregate of tissue exposed to inhaled organisms, a large mass of bacteria, biofilms, can accumulate in the adenoids and cause recurrent infections. Adenoids can be involved in infections of the nose and sinuses.

Symptoms from adenoidal disease are maximal at approximately the age of 6 years. Most adults have minimal amounts of adenoidal tissue; nasopharyngeal masses in adults should be investigated further to exclude other pathology.

Adenoidectomy

Adenoidectomy is a common surgical procedure in children. The main indications for adenoidectomy are as follow:

- Airway obstruction caused by enlarged adenoids (often combined with tonsillectomy in obstructive sleep apnoea)
- OME – as an adjuvant procedure with grommet insertion in recurrent cases of glue ear.

The main contraindications to adenoidectomy are as follow:
- Bleeding disorders
- Palatal abnormalities – the palate must be palpated prior to the procedure to assess for undiagnosed submucosal clefts
- Recent upper respiratory tract infection.

The main complications of adenoidectomy are as follow:
- Bleeding
- Velopharyngeal insufficiency (i.e. nasal regurgitation). This is rare and usually short-lived.
- Hypernasality – can be a significant problem if a patient has undiagnosed palatal deformity. Air escapes from the nose during speech.

Rare nasopharyngeal conditions
Nasopharyngeal cancer

This is rare in Western communities. It is more common in individuals who live in certain provinces of China. Epstein–Barr virus has also been implicated in the aetiology. All nasopharyngeal masses in adults as well as unilateral glue ear must be investigated to exclude nasopharyngeal cancer.

Angiofibroma

This is also known as juvenile nasal angiofibroma. It is a very rare tumour found in adolescent males. It is benign but can be very aggressive with local invasion. Patients typically present with unilateral nasal obstruction and a history of recurrent, often heavy, epistaxis. Because of the vascular nature of these tumours patients can bleed very heavily and a high index of suspicion needs to be maintained for early diagnosis and management.

Clinical practice points

- Not all nasal obstruction in children is caused by adenoids.
- Allergic rhinitis is very common and is often underdiagnosed in children.

23 Pharyngeal infections

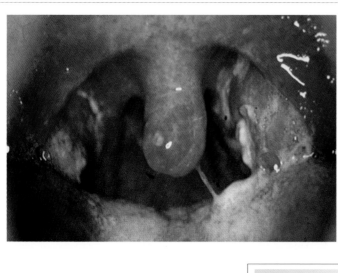

Figure 23.1
Acute tonsillitis
The tonsils are red, swollen and coated with pus. Infectious mononucleosis (glandular fever) has a similar appearance but with a more definite membrane covering the tonsils. The neck nodes will be swollen and tender

Figure 23.2
Outcomes of acute tonsillitis

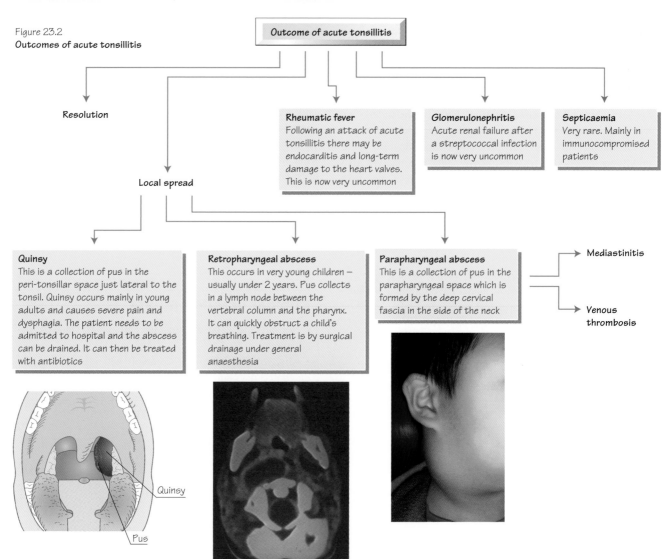

Outcome of acute tonsillitis

Resolution

Rheumatic fever
Following an attack of acute tonsillitis there may be endocarditis and long-term damage to the heart valves. This is now very uncommon

Glomerulonephritis
Acute renal failure after a streptococcal infection is now very uncommon

Septicaemia
Very rare. Mainly in immunocompromised patients

Local spread

Quinsy
This is a collection of pus in the peri-tonsillar space just lateral to the tonsil. Quinsy occurs mainly in young adults and causes severe pain and dysphagia. The patient needs to be admitted to hospital and the abscess can be drained. It can then be treated with antibiotics

Retropharyngeal abscess
This occurs in very young children – usually under 2 years. Pus collects in a lymph node between the vertebral column and the pharynx. It can quickly obstruct a child's breathing. Treatment is by surgical drainage under general anaesthesia

Parapharyngeal abscess
This is a collection of pus in the parapharyngeal space which is formed by the deep cervical fascia in the side of the neck

Mediastinitis

Venous thrombosis

Quinsy

Pus

Ear, Nose and Throat at a Glance, First Edition. Nazia Munir and Ray Clarke.

Aetiology

The pharynx can become acutely infected, usually as a result of a virus. This acute pharyngitis is part of many upper respiratory infections including the common cold – acute coryza. Infection of the pharynx can cause enlargement of the tonsils – acute tonsillitis (Figure 23.1). Acute tonsillitis is one of the most common infections in children and young adults. A typical attack of acute tonsillitis will last from 3 to 7 days. The main organisms implicated are as follow:

- Viruses
- Pyogenic bacteria:
  - *Haemophilus influenzae*
  - *Pneumococcus* spp.
  - Haemolytic *Streptococcus.*

The main clinical features at presentation include the following:

- Sore throat
- Odynophagia (painful swallow)
- Fever
- Malaise
- Enlarged cervical lymph nodes
- Enlarged red tonsils.

Treatment is controversial because viral infection is not influenced by antibiotics and most bacterial infections undergo spontaneous resolution. Many authorities argue that an acute sore throat is adequately treated with good analgesia and liberal fluids. If an on-going significant bacterial infection is suspected, then a short course of antibiotics is sensible. Oral penicillin V is the first line antibiotic of choice. Amoxicillin and ampicillin should be avoided if glandular fever is suspected as the patient may develop a florid rash in response to these antibiotics.

Investigation

If infectious mononucleosis (glandular fever) is suspected then a differential blood count and a glandular fever screen (Paul–Bunnell or monospot blood test) can be helpful. A finding of a raised monocyte count on the white cell differential usually indicates glandular fever even if the glandular fever screen is normal. A full blood count is also useful if there is any suspicion of agranulocytosis – this can be a presentation of leukaemia. Diphtheria is extremely rare, but in parts of the world where it is common then a smear and culture can help to establish the diagnosis.

Complications and outcome

Most cases of acute tonsillitis resolve spontaneously with no ill-effects. However, it can be a serious disease particularly in the immuno-compromised patient (Figure 23.2). Most patients are treated in the community but if they cannot swallow fluids, they may require admission to hospital.

Unusual pharyngeal infections

Chronic pharyngitis can cause constant discomfort in the throat, often with a feeling of dryness and phlegm.

Chronic infections such as syphilis and tuberculosis can also involve the pharynx.

Clinical practice point

Acute tonsillitis is usually benign and self-limiting, but complications – although rare – can be very serious.

24 Tonsillectomy

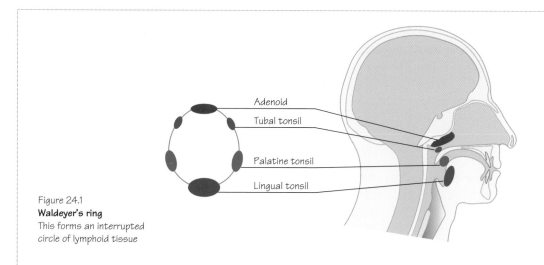

Figure 24.1
Waldeyer's ring
This forms an interrupted circle of lymphoid tissue

Adenoid
Tubal tonsil
Palatine tonsil
Lingual tonsil

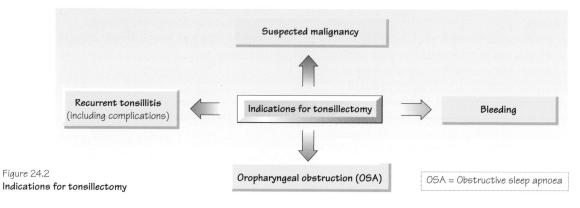

Suspected malignancy

Recurrent tonsillitis
(including complications)

Indications for tonsillectomy

Bleeding

Oropharyngeal obstruction (OSA)

OSA = Obstructive sleep apnoea

Figure 24.2
Indications for tonsillectomy

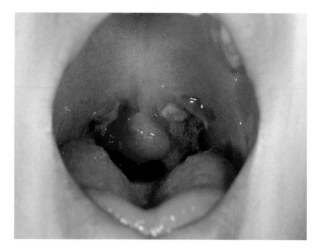

Figure 24.3
The pharynx 2 days after a tonsillectomy
Note the white membrane covering the tonsil beds.
This is normal scar tissue and does not need antibiotics

Tonsils

When we refer to the tonsils we usually mean the collections of lymphoid tissue at the entrance to the pharynx, on either side of the uvula (i.e. the palatine tonsils). There are also lingual tonsils at the base of the tongue. All of these as well as the adenoids are part of Waldeyer's ring (Figure 24.1), which is a collection of lymphoid tissue that forms a circle around the entrance to the upper respiratory tract and forms the first line of defence against infection.

The tonsils are lined with squamous epithelium. This lining forms crypts that extend well into the body of the tonsil, where pus and debris can collect. Tonsils, like adenoids, are especially well developed in children and reduce in size as the child gets older. They can still be large and troublesome in teenagers and young adults, less so in middle-aged and older patients.

Pharyngeal lymphoid tissue is important for developing immunity in very young children. After the age of 2 years this effect seems to tail off, hence surgical removal of the tonsils and adenoids in older children (adenotonsillectomy) has no adverse effect on the child's resistance to infection.

Diseases of the tonsils

Infection of the tonsils is common and one of the most important reasons for antibiotic use. Children and young adults are most susceptible. Most infections are viral and short-lived. Bacterial infections (e.g. streptococcal sore throat) tend to be more severe and last longer, often interfering with the child's schooling or, in the case of adults, causing repeated absences from work (see Chapter 23).

Large tonsils can contribute to airway obstruction, especially in young children (see Chapter 27).

The tonsil can be the site of malignant disease – squamous cell carcinoma of the oropharynx in adults and very rarely lymphoma or rhamdomyosarcoma in children where the presentation may be unilateral tonsil swelling.

Repeated bleeding from the mouth can sometimes be traced to the tonsil (haemorrhagic tonsils) when an area of prominent blood vessels on the surface of the tonsil is the source.

Tonsillectomy

Tonsillectomy is one of the most common operations performed in both adults and children. The indications for tonsillectomy are still controversial (Figure 24.2). About 50,000 tonsillectomies are performed in England and Wales per year, two-thirds of them in children. In children with obstructive sleep apnoea, adenoidectomy is often combined with tonsillectomy, but only if there is an obvious adenoidal enlargement. Tonsillectomy is painful and should only be recommended when well-defined criteria apply.

Recurrent acute tonsillitis is the main reason for removing the tonsils. The Scottish Intercollegiate Guidelines Network (SIGN) recommendations are regularly updated in light of best evidence and provide a good evidence base for clinical practice (www.sign.ac.uk). Current SIGN recommendations for indications for performing tonsillectomy for recurrent sore throats in both children and adults are as follow:
• Sore throats due to acute tonsillitis
• Episodes bad enough to need time off work or school
• Seven or more episodes in 1 year, five or more in 2 consecutive years or three or more in 3 consecutive years.
Other indications for tonsillectomy include suspected malignancy, especially in older patients, and recurrent bleeding from the pharynx.

Tonsillectomy is painful and the patient will need a general anaesthetic for the procedure, a short hospital stay and about 2 weeks off school or work after the procedure. It is normal to have a sloughy appearance of the tonsillar fossae after the operation (Figure 24.3). This slough is not an indication of postoperative infection and therefore does not require antibiotics. The main postoperative complication of both tonsillectomy and adenoidectomy is bleeding.

Clinical practice point

Tonsillectomy is one of the most common operations performed in both adults and children, but the indications remain controversial.

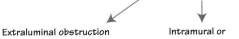

Causes of dysphagia

Extraluminal obstruction
• Neck mass
• Mediastinal mass
• Abnormal blood vessel
  e.g. double aortic arch
  causing 'dysphagia lusoria'

Intramural or neurological causes
• Motor neurone disease
• Multiple sclerosis
• Stroke
• Motility disorders

Intraluminal obstruction
• Foreign body
• Cancer
• Stricture

Figure 25.1
Causes of dysphagia

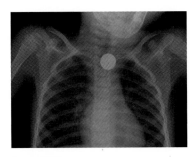

Figure 25.2
X-ray of a coin in the oesophagus

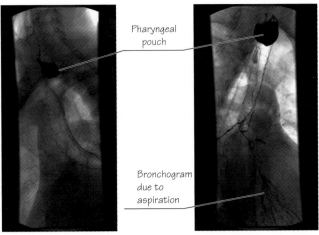

Pharyngeal pouch

Bronchogram due to aspiration

Figure 25.3a
Barium swallow showing pharyngeal pouch
(Note fluid level in the barium filled pouch)

Figure 25.3b
Barium swallow showing a bronchogram due to aspiration of contrast
(same patient as in Figure 25.3a)

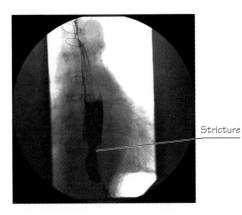

Stricture

Figure 25.4
Barium swallow showing a stricture at the lower end of the oesophagus causing hold up of contrast proximally

Definitions

Dysphagia is difficulty swallowing. Globus is a sensation of a lump in the throat. Odynophagia is pain on swallowing.

Aetiology

Swallowing problems can be caused by obstruction within the pharynx and oesophagus (intraluminal), by external pressure on the pharynx and oesophagus by a neck or mediastinal mass (extraluminal) or by neurological disorders that affect the swallowing muscles (intramural; Figure 25.1). The history should include pertinent questions to help to identify the cause:

• *Degree of dysphagia:* solids, tablets, liquids, saliva.
• *Does the patient have difficulty making the movements of swallowing:* this can help differentiate a physical obstruction from a neurological cause.
• *Level of dysphagia:* in the neck, upper, mid or low chest.
• *Timescale of symptoms:* how long has the patient had symptoms for?
• *Presence of odynophagia:* is there any pain on swallowing?
• *Weight loss:* the amount of weight loss if this can be quantified.
• *Voice change:* hoarseness.
• *Smoking and alcohol history.*
• *Associated symptoms:* including otalgia, regurgitation of food or liquids, other neurological symptoms.

Foreign body

Sharp bones, especially fish bones, can get stuck in the tongue base or in the tonsil. They may be extremely uncomfortable and need to be removed, usually by an ENT surgeon. Children may swallow coins or toys that get stuck at the entrance to the oesophagus at the level of the cricopharynx muscle (Figure 25.2). The child will be distressed, may not be able to swallow and in some cases will have airway obstruction as the object not only blocks the oesophagus, but also presses against the trachea. Adults, especially elderly patients, are more likely to present with a bolus of food, often a piece of poorly chewed meat impacting in the oesophagus. This is again commonly lodged at the cricopharynx. Foreign bodies may pass but, if not, they will need to be removed by rigid oesophagoscopy under a general anaesthetic or by flexible oesophagogastroduodenoscopy (OGD) under sedation. Foreign bodies containing bone, batteries or sharp objects need to be removed urgently because of trauma to the pharynx or oesophagus.

Globus pharyngeus

Globus refers to a sensation of a lump in the throat. Often, the patient will complain of dryness, discomfort in the throat and sometimes of a feeling of pressure when swallowing. The condition used to be known as globus hystericus and was thought to be psychological. There is often a background of anxiety, cancer phobia, work or family-related stress, or a recent illness. Globus affects women more frequently than men and is unusual before the age of about 35 years although it can occur in younger patients including children and adolescents. The pathophysiology of globus is not well understood, but it is thought to be caused by abnormal tension in the cricopharynx muscle that separates the pharynx from the upper oesophagus. Acid reflux into the upper oesophagus and pharynx is also thought have a role. Patients with globus are often extremely anxious and it is wise to refer them to an ENT surgeon for a thorough examination including endoscopy, usually possible in the clinic. Treatment is by reassurance. If there is associated gastroesophageal reflux (GOR) this may also need to be treated.

Investigation of dysphagia

Dysphagia nearly always warrants urgent referral. A barium swallow (Figures 25.3 and 25.4) will help to show a pharyngeal pouch, a stricture or a malignancy. Oesophageal cancer often presents late and treatment is by surgery and/or chemotherapy and radiotherapy. Advanced stage tumours carry a poor prognosis.

Oesophagoscopy is often combined with inspection of the stomach and duodenum – an OGD. This will give a very good view of the oesophageal lumen; however, rigid upper oesophagoscopy provides a better view of the upper third of the oesophagus, pharynx and larynx.

Oesophageal motility disorders include achalasia or cardiospasm and idiopathic oesophageal spasm. The oesophageal muscles are poorly coordinated and close off the lower oesophageal sphincter. These cases are best investigated with dynamic investigations such as video fluoroscopy. Treatment is often with antispasmodics with input from dietitians and the speech and language therapy team to help improve swallowing function.

Swallowing problems in the elderly
Neurological disorders

Stroke, bulbar palsy and motor neurone disease can affect the swallow as there may be poor coordination of the swallow muscles. Patients may cough because of aspiration of fluid or food into the trachea and lungs.

Pharyngeal pouch

This is mainly a problem in the elderly. A pouch of mucosa herniates from the pharyngeal lumen just above the level of the cricopharynx muscle (Figure 25.3a). It occurs because of poor relaxation of the cricopharynx muscle on swallowing. There is often a poor swallow and the patient presents with dysphagia. In the later stages, food can collect in the pouch and may be regurgitated. Patients with a pharyngeal pouch may also experience significant amounts of aspiration (Figure 25.3b). Treatment is surgical and can usually be undertaken endoscopically.

Clinical practice point

Every patient who presents with true dysphagia (i.e. difficulty swallowing) should be referred for urgent assessment.

---

26 The oral cavity and tongue

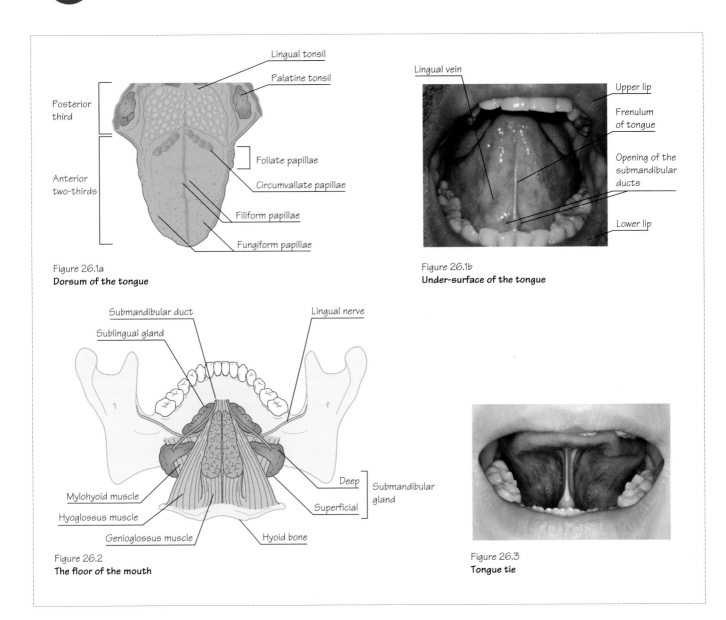

Figure 26.1a
Dorsum of the tongue

Figure 26.1b
Under-surface of the tongue

Figure 26.2
The floor of the mouth

Figure 26.3
Tongue tie

The oral cavity

The oral cavity contains the teeth and gums and the tongue. The tongue is a largely muscular organ that lies on the floor of the mouth (Figure 26.1). The floor of the mouth, although covered with mucosa, is made up mainly of the mylohyoid muscle, stretching from one side of the mandible to the other like a sling (Figure 26.2).

The tongue

The tongue is divided into an anterior two-thirds and a posterior one-third (Figure 26.1a). The posterior third is in the oropharynx and as well as tongue muscle contains collections of lymphoid tissue – the lingual tonsils. These can become enlarged and infected causing trouble with breathing and swallowing.

The tongue contains the taste buds and numerous small salivary glands. The tongue has a very rich blood supply from the lingual artery (Figure 26.1b) and from other branches of the external carotid artery. The motor nerve supply to the tongue is from the hypoglossal nerve. In patients who have had trauma to the hypoglossal nerve, the tongue will deviate to the side ipsilateral to the nerve damage when the tongue is protruded.

The floor of the mouth

The mylohyoid muscle separates the oral cavity from the neck (Figure 26.2). Important structures in the floor of the mouth include the openings of the submandibular ducts that drains saliva from the submandibular glands (Figure 26.2). The sublingual glands are also in this area. The space underneath the mylohyoid is termed the submandibular space. If infection spreads from a dental source, this can cause pus to collect in this area – a submandibular abscess. If this progresses with a spreading cellulitis down the anterior neck it is termed Ludwig's angina. This needs to be treated by broad-spectrum intravenous antibiotics and if it is extensive can compromise the airway and may need surgical drainage and tracheotomy.

Examination

A good light source is paramount for examination of the oral cavity and tongue. A good view of the floor of the mouth can be achieved by asking the patient to move the tongue upwards to the roof of the mouth. Openings of the submandibular ducts should be visible on either side of the midline. The tight band of tissue that connects the tongue to the floor of the mouth is known as the frenulum. This frenulum is tight and short in patients with tongue tie (Figure 26.3). Tongue tie is controversial and many authorities feel that it is an entirely benign condition that does not require treatment. It may interfere with breast feeding in a newborn baby and if so it can be divided easily in a specialist outpatient clinic.

Examination of the oral cavity and tongue is also important as part of the general assessment of a patient with systemic disease. A number of systemic diseases affect the oral mucosa (e.g. jaundice, anaemia and the pigmentation associated with Addison's disease). In acquired immune deficiency syndrome (AIDS) oral candidiasis, or herpetic blisters and Kaposi's sarcoma – a tumour that may present in the gums – can be the mode of presentation.

Mouth ulcers

These are extremely common. They are often idiopathic – aphthous ulcers. Other lesions on the oral mucosa include leukoplakia and erythroplakia – these are white and red patches, respectively, and need careful surveillance as in some cases they can be premalignant.

Clinical practice point

Tongue-tie is common and usually needs no treatment. If it is severe enough to interfere with breast feeding the frenulum can be divided as an outpatient procedure.

Snoring and obstructive sleep apnoea

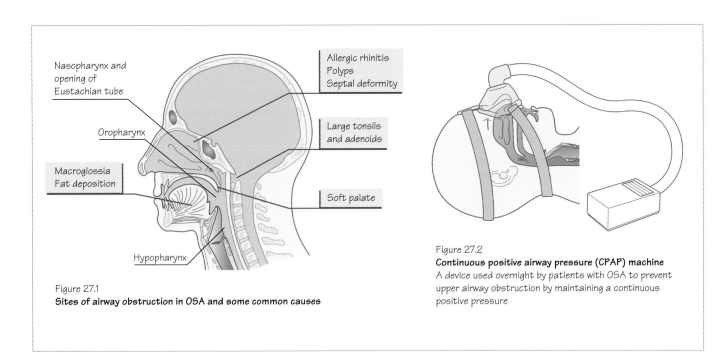

Nasopharynx and opening of Eustachian tube

Oropharynx

Macroglossia
Fat deposition

Hypopharynx

Allergic rhinitis
Polyps
Septal deformity

Large tonsils
and adenoids

Soft palate

Figure 27.1
Sites of airway obstruction in OSA and some common causes

Figure 27.2
Continuous positive airway pressure (CPAP) machine
A device used overnight by patients with OSA to prevent upper airway obstruction by maintaining a continuous positive pressure

Pathophysiology

The pharyngeal muscles relax during sleep causing some degree of airway obstruction as the lumen of the airway reduces in size. Part of the airway can vibrate during inspiration causing snoring. In more serious cases complete closure of the airway causes apnoea, which means air entry stops completely. This is usually very short-lived and the patient wakes up quickly and takes another breath; these are known as arousals. Repeated apnoeas and arousals lead to very poor quality sleep and can have long-term ill effects such as hypertension, increased susceptibility to a stroke and cardiac disease.

About 4% of men and 2% of women have obstructive sleep apnoea (OSA). The main symptoms are snoring, excessive sleepiness during the day and reduced performance at work or, in the case of children, at school. OSA syndrome is thought to be an important factor in road traffic accidents, as severely affected patients can have episodes during the day when driving or operating machinery. In children it can contribute towards problems at school, behavioural issues as well as failure to thrive.

Diagnosis

A thorough history is crucial. Enquire about daytime sleepiness, snoring and the patient's overall sleep pattern. Often, the patient themself will be unaware of the problem and the history will be obtained from a partner. In the case of a child, the parents will sometimes make a video showing the child's sleep pattern, in particular showing the episode of apnoea preceded by the child struggling to breathe and then briefly stopping, before waking up.

It is important to perform a thorough physical examination and in particular to assess the cardiovascular system. In doubtful cases, a specialist sleep clinic will often arrange sleep studies (also known as polysomnography), which may involve an overnight stay. These involve measurement of a number of factors including pulse oximetry, eye movement, brain activity, muscle activity and heart rhythm.

Causes
Adults

Any pathology that gives rise to nasal or pharyngeal airway obstruction can unmask a tendency to OSA (Figure 27.1). Obesity is a major factor in adults, probably because of deposition of adipose tissue in the airway and in the neck. Other important factors are alcohol and cigarette smoking. Men are more likely to develop OSA than women, probably because of the different deposition pattern of adipose tissue in obesity. Hormonal factors can also come into play and OSA can present in women, especially after the menopause.

Children

This is most often caused by enlarged tonsils and adenoids. Mild cases can be treated by observation. More serious cases need to be referred to an ENT surgeon for an adenotonsillectomy. Children with Down syndrome and those with cerebral palsy are especially susceptible. Pharyngeal muscle hypotonia can be implicated in these cases.

Effects

Repeated hypoxia brought about by the apnoeic episodes can have serious long-term effects on the cardiovascular system. OSA is also an important cause of poor performance at work. In children, prolonged OSA can cause failure to thrive. Patients with a definite diagnosis of OSA must inform the Driver and Vehicle Licensing Agency (DVLA).

Treatment
Conservative treatment

Treatment involves addressing the underlying cause or managing the episodes of apnoea. If the patient is obese, then a weight loss management program should be undertaken. Advice regarding alcohol consumption and smoking is also essential. If there is an obvious cause of airway obstruction – such as nasal polyps, nasal septal deviation – these need to be managed concurrently.

Continuous positive airway pressure (CPAP; Figure 27.2) This involves using a face mask that emits a continuing stream of air to keep the airway open during the patient's sleep. This is sometimes referred to as a pneumatic splint. CPAP machines are not always well tolerated, but can be very effective.

Surgery

Surgery is rarely needed for snoring and OSA in adults, but a variety of techniques have been tried. This includes various procedures to stiffen the wall of the pharynx, to remove part of the palate or to reduce the size of the tongue base. In very severe cases, surgery can be used to reconstruct the maxilla and mandible to widen the air passages. All of these procedures are highly specialised and the outcome is uncertain. In paediatric cases, however, adenotonsillectomy is especially effective.

Clinical practice point

Obesity is the main feature in the aetiology of OSA in adults and weight reduction is the most important aspect of management.

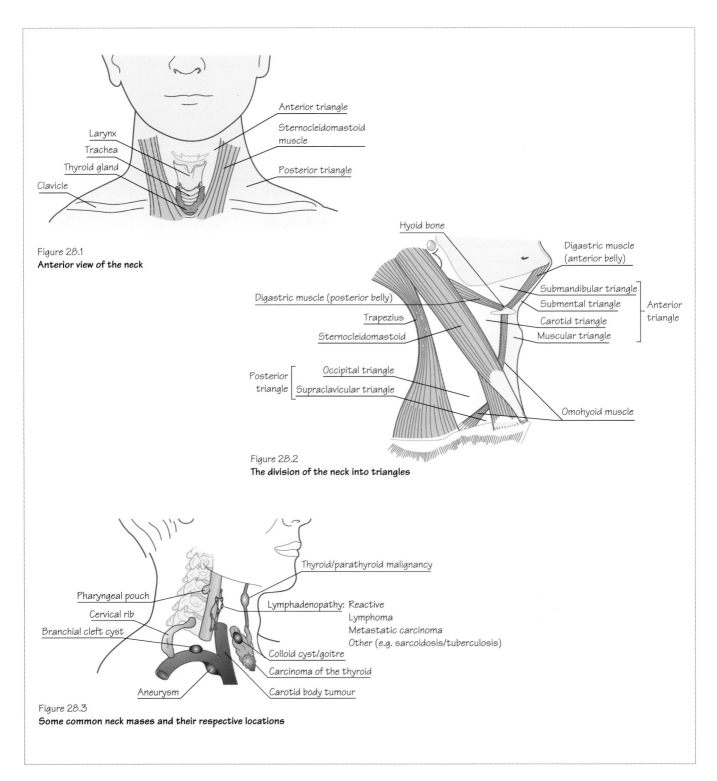

Figure 28.1
Anterior view of the neck

Anterior triangle
Sternocleidomastoid muscle
Posterior triangle
Larynx
Trachea
Thyroid gland
Clavicle

Hyoid bone
Digastric muscle (anterior belly)
Digastric muscle (posterior belly)
Trapezius
Sternocleidomastoid
Submandibular triangle
Submental triangle
Carotid triangle
Muscular triangle
Anterior triangle
Posterior triangle
Occipital triangle
Supraclavicular triangle
Omohyoid muscle

Figure 28.2
The division of the neck into triangles

Pharyngeal pouch
Cervical rib
Branchial cleft cyst
Aneurysm
Thyroid/parathyroid malignancy
Lymphadenopathy: Reactive
Lymphoma
Metastatic carcinoma
Other (e.g. sarcoidosis/tuberculosis)
Colloid cyst/goitre
Carcinoma of the thyroid
Carotid body tumour

Figure 28.3
Some common neck mases and their respective locations

Anatomy

The neck is separated from the face and head above by the mandible in front and the skull (occipital bone) behind. Below, it becomes the thorax at the clavicles and the first rib. It is neatly separated into anterior and posterior triangles by the sternocleidomastoid muscle (Figure 28.1). It is further subdivided into other triangles (Figure 28.2).

The main structures in the midline of the neck are the pharynx and oesophagus, and the larynx and trachea. These form part of a combined upper aero-digestive tract connecting the nose and mouth above to the lungs and the stomach and gastrointestinal tract below. The main vascular supply of the head and brain – the carotid arteries and the jugular veins – run in the neck lateral to the midline in the carotid sheath which lies beneath the sternocleidomastoid muscle. The vagus nerve (the tenth cranial nerve) also runs in the carotid sheath with the major vessels from the brain to the chest. The thyroid and the parathyroid glands are found lower in the anterior neck, with the major salivary glands (parotid, submandibular and sublingual glands) in the upper neck. The neck also contains the lower cranial nerves and the phrenic nerve which arises from cervical nerves 3–5 and innervates the diaphragm.

Fascia and spaces Most of the structures of the neck are surrounded by a series of dense layers of connective tissue know as fascia. These form tight capsules around the parotid glands and the thyroid gland and merge with the carotid sheaths on either side of the neck. Important spaces are formed within these fascial planes, most notably the parapharyngeal space just lateral to the pharynx. This is an area where infection and pus can collect giving rise to a parapharyngeal abscess (see Chapter 23).

Lymph nodes The neck contains over a hundred lymph nodes. These are found in both the anterior and posterior triangle but form a number of discreet groups of glands (see Chapter 29). They can become enlarged due to a number of causes including infection and malignancy.

Examination of the neck

Exposure should be adequate down to the level of the clavicle and neck jewellery should be removed.

Inspection

Evaluation commences with inspection of the patient as a whole for any peripheral stigmata of disease. The neck is evaluated at rest and on swallowing from the front; this is best accomplished by giving the patient a sip of water rather than a dry swallow – neck masses may become more obvious on swallowing. Asymmetry, neck masses and their location, skin colour and changes, swelling and neck scars should be inspected.

Palpation

Palpation of the lump should take place from behind the seated patient with their head and neck slightly flexed. A systematic approach to palpation is essential in order to assess the whole of the neck – patients who present with a specific neck lump may have other palpable masses. Palpation is performed using the pulp of the fingers not the tips to best assess the nature of any lesions. One technique is to start palpating under the chin to feel the submental nodes, working backwards under the jaw to feel the submandibular area (including the submandibular salivary glands) back to the angle of the jaw and the jugulodigastric or tonsillar nodes. Palpation proceeds down along the sternomastoid muscles to feel for any nodes in the deep cervical chain down to the suprasternal notch. The trachea, thyroid and central neck including the larynx are palpated up to and including the hyoid bone. The neck is then palpated working out laterally above the clavicles, up into the posterior triangle and along the border of the trapezius muscles up to the mastoid and occipital regions. Finally, both parotid glands are felt for any masses.

The position, size and consistency of any neck masses should be assessed. The mobility and fixity of the mass to overlying and adjacent structures should also be looked for. Pulsatile masses suggest a vascular origin and fluctuant masses suggest a fluid-filled or cystic lesion – it may be helpful to transilluminate these masses. Large cysts will typically transilluminate, but this is a fairly insensitive sign. Figure 28.3 illustrates some differential diagnoses of neck lumps and their typical positions in the neck. Percussion of the chest to assess for retrosternal extension is carried out for suspected thyroid masses and auscultation of the mass is performed to assess for a bruit.

Clinical practice points

- The sternocleidomastoid muscle is the key to the anatomy of the neck.
- A systematic and thorough approach to examination of the neck is essential.
- The order of examination should be inspection, palpation, percussion, auscultation.
- Correlation of any masses should be made with the normal structures found in the region of the neck being examined.

29 Neck lumps

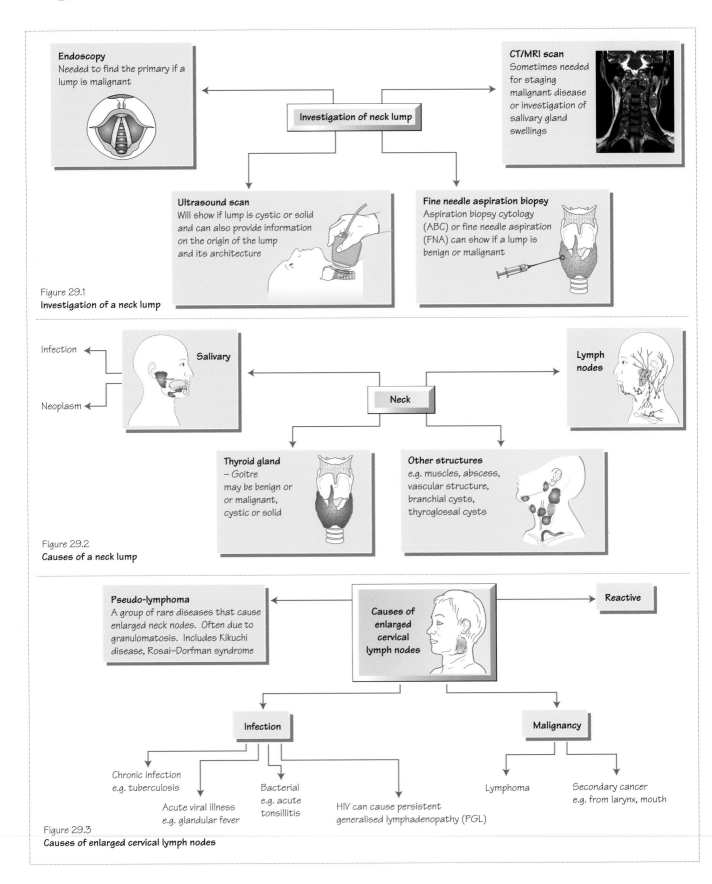

Endoscopy
Needed to find the primary if a lump is malignant

CT/MRI scan
Sometimes needed for staging malignant disease or investigation of salivary gland swellings

Investigation of neck lump

Ultrasound scan
Will show if lump is cystic or solid and can also provide information on the origin of the lump and its architecture

Fine needle aspiration biopsy
Aspiration biopsy cytology (ABC) or fine needle aspiration (FNA) can show if a lump is benign or malignant

Figure 29.1
Investigation of a neck lump

Infection

Neoplasm

Salivary

Neck

Lymph nodes

Thyroid gland
– Goitre may be benign or or malignant, cystic or solid

Other structures
e.g. muscles, abscess, vascular structure, branchial cysts, thyroglossal cysts

Figure 29.2
Causes of a neck lump

Pseudo-lymphoma
A group of rare diseases that cause enlarged neck nodes. Often due to granulomatosis. Includes Kikuchi disease, Rosai–Dorfman syndrome

Causes of enlarged cervical lymph nodes

Reactive

Infection

Malignancy

Chronic infection e.g. tuberculosis

Acute viral illness e.g. glandular fever

Bacterial e.g. acute tonsillitis

HIV can cause persistent generalised lymphadenopathy (PGL)

Lymphoma

Secondary cancer e.g. from larynx, mouth

Figure 29.3
Causes of enlarged cervical lymph nodes

Ear, Nose and Throat at a Glance, First Edition. Nazia Munir and Ray Clarke.
66 © 2013 Nazia Munir and Ray Clarke. Published 2013 by Blackwell Publishing Ltd.

A lump in the neck is a common clinical problem. Most neck lumps are benign, but differentiation from lesions that could be malignant is vital. Therefore, a sensible, structured approach is required to assess and evaluate each patient to decide who can simply be reassured and who requires further investigation and referral for a specialist opinion.

Evaluation

All approaches to a neck lump begin with a thorough and complete history of the lump, including the site, chronicity, aggravating and relieving factors, lumps in other body sites, pain and discharge from the lump. A full ENT and head and neck history is mandatory, ensuring 'red flag' symptoms are asked about:

- Hoarseness (persisting for more than 3 weeks)
- Dysphagia
- Odynophagia (painful swallow)
- Unexplained otalgia
- Non-healing ulcers
- White or red patches in the mouth or oropharynx
- Facial or cheek swelling
- Unexplained loosening of teeth.

The history should also include information on systemic symptoms including the following:

- Weight loss
- Night sweats
- Lethargy and tiredness.

Past medical and surgical, drug and family history should be taken. Importantly, smoking and alcohol use should be documented as well as other pertinent social history.

Examination should include the lump in the context of the rest of the head and neck (see Chapter 28). A full ENT examination is also undertaken assessing the upper aero-digestive tract. Axillary, abdominal and groin examination should be performed if nodes are present in these sites.

Investigations

Investigation of the mass should be to confirm or refute the suspected diagnosis. As with breast masses, triple assessment comprising of clinical, radiological and cytological evaluation is needed (Figure 29.1). Radiology and cytology are often combined by performing an ultrasound-guided fine needle aspiration (FNA). Use of the ultrasound allows the mass in question and the rest of the neck to be identified and characterised as well as accurately guiding the needle for the FNA. Ultrasound-guided FNA is more likely to yield a positive and representative sample of the mass in question. Further radiological assessment with magnetic resonance imaging (MRI) or computed tomography (CT) scanning is sometimes required for further characterisation of the mass or of the primary lesion in the case of malignancy. Upper aero-digestive tract endoscopy under general anaesthetic might be required after the above investigations, again to evaluate a primary lesion in the case of malignancy. Neck nodes should *not* be excised without a full diagnostic work-up as this may compromise disease management in cancer cases. Referral to a specialist head and neck clinic should take place for further management, especially in the case of diagnostic difficulties.

Aetiology

Figure 29.2 illustrates the common causes of a neck lump. Use of a surgical sieve approach can help to identify the cause of the neck lump. Generally, they can be divided into nodal masses and non-nodal masses.

Non-nodal masses

Thyroid masses

The thyroid gland sits in the anterior neck (like a bow tie) overlying the trachea. It is adherent to the trachea by the pre-tracheal fascia; this is a condensation of the connective tissue in the neck overlying the windpipe. As a result, thyroid masses characteristically move on swallowing – as the larynx and trachea move up and down, so too does the thyroid gland. Thyroid masses are common in adults but rare in children. They are best assessed radiologically with an ultrasound scan and FNA to obtain a tissue sample to identify the nature of the lump. Further details of thyroid masses and disease can be found in Chapter 36.

Salivary masses

Parotid masses can be located in the main body of the gland or in the tail – this is the portion of the gland that is posterior and inferior to the angle of the mandible. Submandibular and parotid tail masses can be primary salivary lesions or lymph nodes, hence careful clinical examination alongside ultrasound and FNA will help to differentiate between the two. Further details of salivary masses and disease can be found in Chapter 35.

Cystic neck masses

Children and young adults may present with a cystic swelling in the middle of the neck. Patients may simply notice the lump, or may attend because of infection in the cyst. Clinically, these lumps move when the patient swallows and on sticking out their tongue and are likely to be a thyroglossal duct cyst. The thyroglossal duct is the tract along which the thyroid gland descends during embryonic development which fails to obliterate (see Chapter 36). Treatment for this is surgical excision including the central portion of the hyoid bone – known as Sistrunk's procedure. Removal of the bone lessens the chance of recurrence of the cyst after surgery.

Branchial cysts are lateral neck swellings usually seen in young adults arising anterior to the upper third of the sterno-cleidomastoid muscle. Patients present after noticing the mass or because of acute swelling often caused by infection within the mass. The cysts are thought to be due to degeneration within lymph nodes. Clinically, they are firm swellings in the upper neck, which are easy to palpate the front but difficult to feel the posterior extent clearly. FNA will aspirate cloudy cyst contents which may contain cholesterol crystals. Treatment is surgical removal.

In patients over 40 years cystic lumps that clinically resemble branchial cyst should be viewed with suspicion, as metastatic head and neck cancer can present with cystic neck nodes. These should not be removed, but referred on for a specialist head and neck surgical opinion.

Vascular masses

Vascular neck masses are uncommon and are usually related to the carotid artery. These may take the form of abnormal dilatations of the carotid artery (an aneurysm) or a normal but tortuous artery. The carotid bulb (the point at which the internal carotid originates from the common carotid) may be enlarged but normal – this may be mistaken for a vascular mass. Furthermore, a normal lymph node overlying the carotid bifurcation can resemble a vascular lesion. True vascular masses develop at the bifurcation of the common carotid and are called carotid body tumours. These are benign lesions that arise from chemoreceptors in the carotid bulb and present as painless lumps. These are investigated with ultrasound and MRI scans; FNA is generally avoided in these masses. Treatment is by embolisation of the feeding vessels and surgical excision.

Nodal masses

Reactive

Reactive enlargement of lymph nodes refers to the response of lymph nodes to a process (usually inflammatory) within the body. Lymph nodes have a role in the body's immune response; therefore, anything that causes this to be up-regulated can cause nodes to increase in size. This can occur locally in the head and neck or as a systemic phenomenon. A good history can often work out the cause for the enlarged gland and ultrasound appearances are characteristic.

Infective

Infective nodes generally arise from viral or bacterial infections. Viral infections include the common cold, influenza virus, glandular fever (Epstein–Barr virus) and, importantly, HIV. Bacterial infections include tonsillitis, quinsy and chronic infections such as TB (see Figure 29.3). Treatment is supportive for viral infections (i.e. analgesia, anti-inflammatories and adequate fluid intake). Bacterial infections additionally require targeted antibiotic treatment – viral infections do not.

Malignant

Malignant neck nodes can arise as a result of a primary haematological malignancy (lymphoma) or metastatic disease. Lymphoma can present with nodes in the head and neck or with multiple nodes in other areas (axilla, groin, abdomen), as well as enlargement of the liver and spleen. It is often accompanied by type B symptoms, namely weight loss, night sweats and general pruritus (itching). Metastatic nodes arise from spread of cancer from head and neck structures, hence a complete and through head and neck examination is mandatory. However, metastatic nodes can arise from structures below the clavicles, such as the breasts, lungs and abdomen.

Clinical practice point

Lymph node swelling in the neck is common in children and young adults. In older patients especially, an enlarged neck node may be a cancer and the patient needs urgent referral to a head and neck clinic.

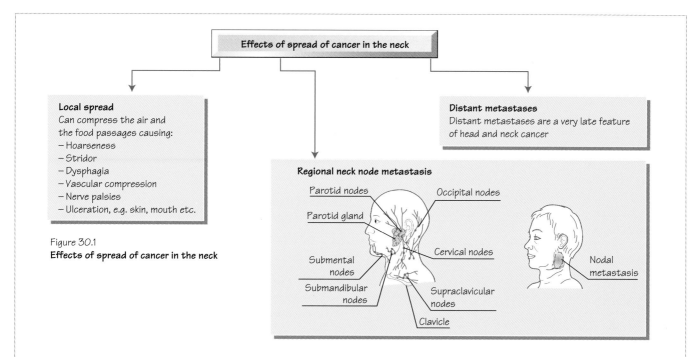

Effects of spread of cancer in the neck

Local spread
Can compress the air and
the food passages causing:
- Hoarseness
- Stridor
- Dysphagia
- Vascular compression
- Nerve palsies
- Ulceration, e.g. skin, mouth etc.

Figure 30.1
Effects of spread of cancer in the neck

Regional neck node metastasis

Parotid nodes
Parotid gland
Submental nodes
Submandibular nodes
Occipital nodes
Cervical nodes
Supraclavicular nodes
Clavicle
Nodal metastasis

Distant metastases
Distant metastases are a very late feature
of head and neck cancer

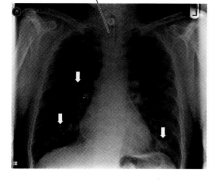

Tracheostomy tube

Figure 30.2
Lung metastasis
Chest X-ray showing multiple lung metastasis
arising from head and neck cancer (some are
highlighted with white arrows). Also note
tracheostomy tube in situ visible on X-ray

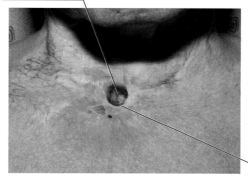

Speech valve in-situ

Laryngectomy stoma

Figure 30.3
Post-laryngectomy patient
The patient breathes through a stoma (hole) in the neck.
Note 'speech valve' present to help with voice rehabilitation
in the absence of a larynx (voice box)

Epidemiology

Cancer of the mucosal surfaces of the upper aero-digestive tract is much less common than lung, breast, colorectal or prostatic cancer, but still an important cause of morbidity and death worldwide. Head and neck squamous cell carcinoma (SCC) accounts for approximately 2600 cancer deaths in the UK annually. It is mainly a disease of men and is more common in the middle aged and elderly. Life style factors are especially important in the aetiology of this type of cancer. Tobacco and excessive alcohol consumption are the two main predisposing factors, each increasing the risk of development of head and neck cancer. However, in patients who both smoke and drink, the risk of getting cancer is more than the sum of the individual risks of each pre-disposing factor (i.e. the risk is multiplicative rather than additive). There is an increasing trend of development of oropharyngeal tumours in a much younger cohort of patients. This is thought to be related to human papilloma virus incidence. Other risk factors include smokeless tobacco (betel nut chewing or snuff) and poor diet.

Histology

Histologically, the predominant type of head and neck cancer is SCC.

Site and spread

The oral cavity is the most common site where SCC develops, followed by the larynx, oropharynx and hypopharynx in descending frequency. Within the oral cavity, tumours arise from the anterior two-thirds of the tongue, floor of the mouth, the gums, hard palate and buccal mucosa (the mucosa over the inner lining of the cheek). Larynx tumours are subdivided into those at the glottis (the level of the vocal cords), supraglottis (above the vocal cords) and subglottis (below the level of the vocal cords). The oropharynx includes the tonsils, soft palate and the base of the tongue, and the hypopharynx consists of the pyriform fossae down to the beginning of the oesophagus. Head and neck tumours also arise in the nose and sinuses and nasopharynx. Skin cancers that arise in the head and neck are not normally classed as head and neck tumours. As with most tumours, head and neck cancer can invade local structures, spread to regional lymph nodes and systemically to the rest of the body (Figure 30.1). Tumours tend to spread to regional neck nodes along relatively predictable pathways – the location of these nodes can often help to identify the location of the primary tumour.

Presentation

It is important to detect these cancers as early as possible, but very often the patient will not present until there has been considerable local invasion or spread to neck nodes. This is especially true in certain head and neck sites such as the supra or sub glottis and hypopharynx, as the patient may experience few or no symptoms until late in the disease process. Some common modes of presentation ('red flag' symptoms) that warrant urgent referral to an ENT surgeon include the following:

- Hoarseness (persisting for more than 3 weeks)
- Dysphagia
- Odynophagia
- Unexplained otalgia
- Neck lump
- Non-healing ulcers of the oral cavity or oropharynx for more than 3 weeks
- White or red patches in the mouth or oropharynx for more than 3 weeks
- Stridor
- Facial or cheek swelling.

Treatment and prognosis

Patients with head and neck SCC are managed within a multidisciplinary team including:

- Head and neck surgeons (ENT and maxillofacial)
- Oncologists
- Radiologists
- Plastic surgeons
- Oral and dental surgeons
- Speech and language therapists
- Dietitians
- Head and neck nurse specialists
- Physiotherapists.

The treatment options include:

- Surgery (open and/or endoscopic)
- Radiotherapy
- Chemotherapy
- Palliative and symptomatic care.

Treatment is tailored to each individual patient and may involve a single modality or be multimodality depending on the site and stage of the disease as well as other factors such as the patient's overall health and well-being and patient choice.

The outcome for head and neck cancer, like most other malignancies, is very good if the disease is caught at the early stages. However, most patients present late when the disease has progressed to an advanced stage. Prognosis is based on the size and degree of local invasion of the primary lesion (the more locally advanced the primary tumour, the worse the survival), presence of spread to local neck nodes (presence of neck metastases reduces long-term survival rates) and distant spread (Figure 30.2). Distant metastases are usually a sign of advanced disease and so poor prognosis.

Rehabilitation

Surgery for head and neck cancer can be mutilating (Figure 30.3). The patient may lose the larynx, part of the pharynx or even a large part of the tongue. This can affect breathing, swallowing and speech. Chemotherapy and radiotherapy can also result in similar long-term problems affecting day to day activities. Patients need very intensive support to help restore these functions and may not gain these back completely. Head and neck cancer surgeons work closely with speech and language therapists, prosthetists and other health care professionals within the multidisciplinary team to ensure optimum care for these patients.

Clinical practice point

Refer patients with 'red flag' symptoms in the head and neck for an urgent ENT opinion.

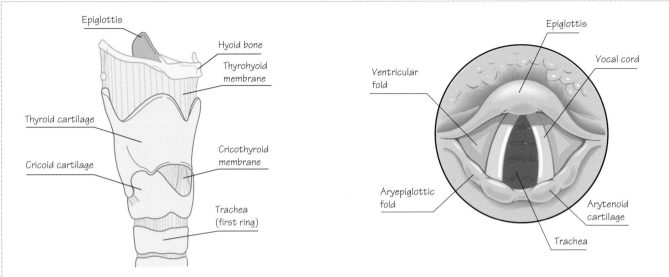

Figure 31.1
Cartilages and membranes of the larynx

Figure 31.2
The vocal cords and trachea from above as seen through a rigid endoscope

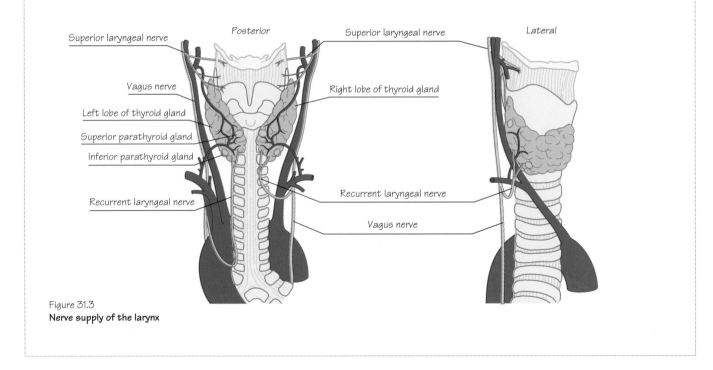

Figure 31.3
Nerve supply of the larynx

Ear, Nose and Throat at a Glance, First Edition. Nazia Munir and Ray Clarke.

72 © 2013 Nazia Munir and Ray Clarke. Published 2013 by Blackwell Publishing Ltd.

Anatomy

The larynx is part of the upper respiratory tract and connects the nasal and pharyngeal air passages to the trachea. It is lined with ciliated columnar epithelium for the most part but some areas – especially the vocal cords or folds – are lined with a tougher keratinised squamous epithelium. The larynx is made up of a series of cartilages joined by membranes and muscles and contains the vocal cords (Figures 31.1 and 31.2). The largest cartilage in the larynx is the thyroid cartilage, which is divided into a left and right lamina. These joint at the front like the keel of a ship and at the uppermost point form the laryngeal prominence or Adam's apple. The thyroid cartilage acts as protection for the vocal cords. Between the thyroid cartilage and the first tracheal ring is the cricoid cartilage. This is a signet ring shaped structure and is the only complete ring in the airway. This is the narrowest point of the upper airway in children whereas the level of the vocal cords is the narrowest point in the adult upper airway. The cricoid cartilage articulates with the thyroid cartilage as well as smaller cartilages within the larynx to allow vocal cord movement and hence voice production. The larynx is attached to the hyoid bone by muscles and membranes which in turn suspend the hyoid bone from the mandible. The muscles that attach to the external part of the larynx elevate and depress the organ during speech and swallowing, these are termed the strap muscles.

Nerve supply The nerves that supply the muscles of the larynx are the superior and recurrent laryngeal nerves. Both are branches of the vagus nerve (Figure 31.3). The recurrent laryngeal nerve branches off the main trunk of the vagus, loops round the aortic arch on the left and the subclavian artery on the right (hence the name **recurrent** laryngeal nerve). It then ascends the neck in the groove between the oesophagus and the trachea to enter the larynx. Here, it supplies the majority of the muscles in the voice box; the superior laryngeal nerve only supplies the cricothyroid muscle which allows pitch alteration in the voice. As a result a patient with lung cancer or a tumour in the mediastinum may develop hoarseness because of vocal cord palsy. The recurrent laryngeal nerves are also closely related to the thyroid and parathyroid glands and are therefore at risk from thyroid malignancies or during thyroid and/or parathyroid surgery.

Lymphatic drainage This is very important in clinical practice. The superior and inferior deep cervical lymph nodes receive lymphatic drainage from the larynx so a patient with laryngeal cancer may develop an enlarged neck node as the cancer spreads. The outlook is much better if the patient can be treated before this spread occurs.

Physiology

The functions of the larynx are related to its special position at the junction between the digestive and the respiratory systems and are threefold:

1 To allow air in and out of the lungs (respiration)
2 To produce voice (phonation)
3 To protect the airways during swallowing (aspiration).

Phonation The intricate arrangement and fine movements of its laryngeal muscles alter the air flow pattern through the larynx and allow the vocal cords to function in much the same way as the reed in a musical instrument. The sound is then modified by the mouth and pharynx to produce the variations in pitch and harmonies that we know as speech. One of the earliest presentations of laryngeal disease is with change in voice (dysphonia).

Protection of the lower airway During swallowing the larynx closes off as the vocal cords move together by reflex contraction. The epiglottis tips backwards, but this is less important. One of the most important factors in prevention of aspiration is laryngeal elevation. The movement of the larynx comes from the strap muscles contracting against the hyoid bone which contracts against the mandible. In a vocal cord palsy where one or more of the cords is paralysed, the patient may not be able to protect their airway and may cough and splutter during swallowing, resulting in food going 'down the wrong way', known as aspiration.

Assessment of the larynx in the ENT clinic

A thorough history enquiring about each of the following symptoms is crucial:
• *Hoarseness:* dysphonia – complete voice loss is termed aphonia
• *Stridor:* partial obstruction of the airway can cause this high-pitched noise to progress to complete airway obstruction
• *Cough:* is there any coughing up of blood?
• *Choking:* on eating and drinking
• *Dysphagia:* difficulty swallowing.

Examination should include a systematic neck and oral cavity examination. The larynx can be visualised using indirect laryngoscopy. In this technique, a good view of the larynx can be gained in cooperative patients using a headlight and a mirror placed against the lower end of the soft palate. The type of view seen in this technique is shown in Figure 31.2. This should not be carried out in patients with compromised airways. However, flexible fibreoptic endoscopy is now the standard method of assessing the larynx in the ENT outpatient clinic, providing an excellent and reliable direct view of the larynx.

Clinical practice points

• If laryngeal symptoms persist, refer the patient to an ENT surgeon for flexible endoscopic assessment.
• Stridor is a very serious sign and can rapidly progress to complete airway obstruction.

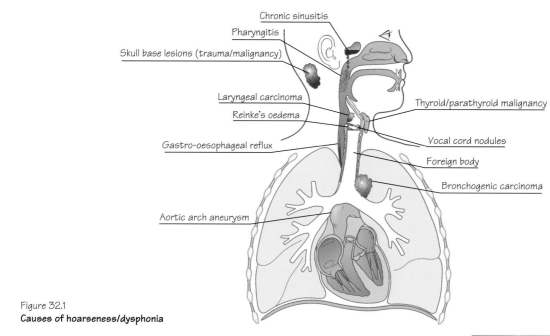

Figure 32.1
Causes of hoarseness/dysphonia

- Chronic sinusitis
- Pharyngitis
- Skull base lesions (trauma/malignancy)
- Laryngeal carcinoma
- Reinke's oedema
- Gastro-oesophageal reflux
- Aortic arch aneurysm
- Thyroid/parathyroid malignancy
- Vocal cord nodules
- Foreign body
- Bronchogenic carcinoma

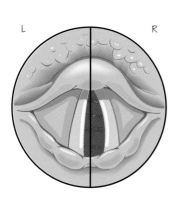

L   R

Figure 32.2
Left vocal cord palsy
The patient has been asked to say
'eeeeeeee' and the right cord has
moved laterally but the left is immobile

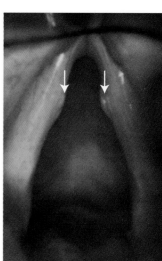

Figure 32.3
Vocal cord nodules
White arrows point to the nodules

Hoarseness

Hoarseness (dysphonia) is a subjective alteration in voice quality. There are many causes of hoarseness (Figure 32.1). Common causes include laryngitis, vocal cord nodules and muscle tension dysphonia. If hoarseness persists for more than 3 weeks it may be secondary to a malignancy and needs referral for specialist ENT assessment.

Acute laryngitis

This is a common feature of upper respiratory tract infections and can last up to 2 weeks. Treatment is with fluids, analgesia and anti-inflammatory drugs. Voice rest should be encouraged during the acute phase, especially avoidance of whispering, shouting and forcing the voice.

Chronic laryngitis

Smoking, alcohol and excessive or misuse of the voice, for example in professional voice users (e.g. teachers, actors) can cause chronic inflammation. Advise voice rest and smoking cessation. For prolonged symptoms get the help of a speech and language therapist (SALT). In smokers, chronic laryngitis can progress to dysplasia, then carcinoma *in situ* and finally invasive carcinoma.

Vocal cord palsy

Hoarseness, and in some cases aspiration, can be caused by inability of one or both of the cords to appose (Figure 32.2). The laryngeal muscles are mainly supplied by the recurrent laryngeal nerves, branches of the vagus nerve. Any pathology that affects these nerves can cause hoarseness. Causes of vocal cord paralysis include trauma to the nerve, which may be iatrogenic (i.e. after thyroid or parathyroid surgery), a mediastinal mass (e.g. bronchogenic carcinoma) and thyroid malignancy.

Vocal cord nodules

Repeated trauma to the edge of the cords – typically caused by excessive or untutored voice projection – can cause submucosal fibrosis and the development of nodules (Figure 32.3). Voice rest and SALT are usually all that are needed. Vocal cord nodules are also see in children as a cause for hoarseness; treatment is the same.

Muscle tension dysphonia

Voice problems can be caused by incoordination of the laryngeal muscles. SALT assessment and exercises are the main management of this disorder.

Clinical practice points

• Laryngeal cancer typically presents with hoarseness. Be vigilant about early referral and assessment of hoarseness that persists for more than 2–3 weeks.
• The management of voice disorders has improved greatly with the development of specialist voice clinics, usually involving an ENT surgeon and a speech and language therapist (SALT).

See Chapter 31.

33 Acute airway obstruction

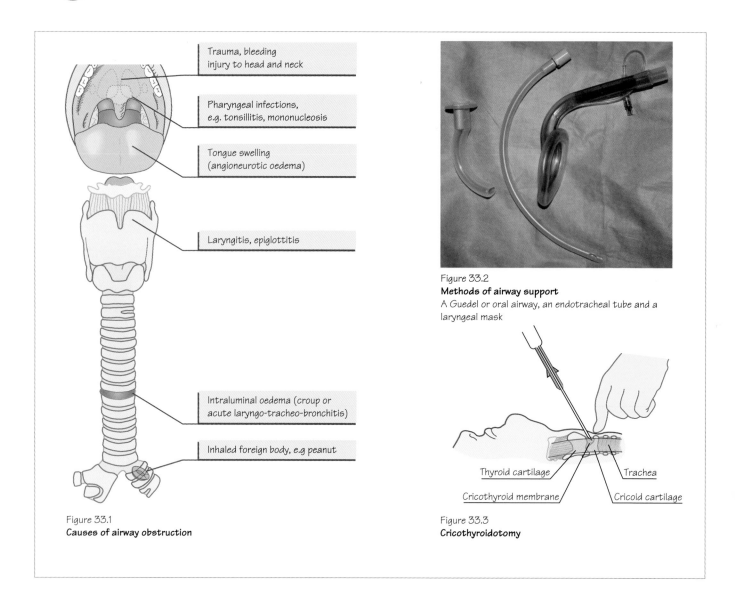

Trauma, bleeding
injury to head and neck

Pharyngeal infections,
e.g. tonsillitis, mononucleosis

Tongue swelling
(angioneurotic oedema)

Laryngitis, epiglottitis

Intraluminal oedema (croup or
acute laryngo-tracheo-bronchitis)

Inhaled foreign body, e.g peanut

Figure 33.1
Causes of airway obstruction

Figure 33.2
Methods of airway support
A Guedel or oral airway, an endotracheal tube and a
laryngeal mask

Thyroid cartilage

Trachea

Cricothyroid membrane

Cricoid cartilage

Figure 33.3
Cricothyroidotomy

The airway extends from the nasal and oral cavities to the alveoli (Figure 33.1). Chronic airway obstruction usually involves the bronchi and the smaller air passages (e.g. chronic obstructive pulmonary disease, COPD). It is essential to recognise and promptly deal with acute obstruction of the larger airways (e.g. the larynx and trachea). Obstruction can be partial or complete. Complete airway obstruction is rapidly fatal but partial airway obstruction is more common. If a severe obstruction is not relieved or bypassed the patient will become hypoxaemic, acidotic and will quickly progress to cardiac arrest, brainstem ischaemia and death.

Some of the causes of airway obstruction are shown in Figure 33.1.

Some of the clinical features of airway obstruction are non-specific. Partial airway obstruction is usually associated with noisy breathing. **Stridor** is a high-pitched noise caused by turbulent flow in the larynx and upper trachea. **Stertor** is a lower pitched noise – much like snoring – associated with pharyngeal obstruction, and usually worse when the patient is asleep as the pharyngeal muscle tone is reduced and vibrates with respiratory activity.

Clinical features of an acutely obstructed airway

- Noisy breathing (stertor or stridor)
- Agitation
- Confusion
- Cyanosis (a late and dangerous sign)
- Tachycardia
- Increased respiratory rate (tachypnoea)
- Unconsciousness
- Sternal recession: the sternum sinks well into the chest during inspiration, most marked in babies because of the softness of the bones in the chest wall
- Tracheal tug: the trachea moves down in the neck during inspiration, especially in children

Management

The most important aspect of management is to make sure the patient has a patent airway, either by removing the obstruction or establishing an alternative air passage. Some 'alternative' airways are shown in Figure 33.2.

- **Guedel** or oral airway is a useful way to keep the tongue base forward in an unconscious patient.
- An **endotracheal** airway is introduced through the mouth or the nose and guided into the trachea via the larynx. This is a skilled and often life-saving procedure (endotracheal intubation).
- **Laryngeal mask airway**, also introduced through the nose or mouth, so that the mask rests on the laryngeal inlet permitting ventilation of the airway.
- An emergency tracheotomy is nowadays very rarely needed, but in an extreme emergency it may be possible to perforate the membrane between the thyroid cartilage and the cricoid cartilage (**cricothyroidotomy**; Figure 33.3).

Non-specific measures helpful in managing airway obstruction

- *Oxygen therapy:* will not overcome obstruction but can prevent hypoxia in the short term.
- *Adrenaline:* nebulised adrenaline can help to open the small airways in particular, but the effect is temporary.
- *Steroids:* oral prednisolone or dexamethasone can reduce airway mucosal oedema.

Clinical practice points

- The most important measure in managing acute airway obstruction is to remove the obstruction. If you cannot do this, try to establish an alternative airway until the patient can have definitive treatment.
- In suspected airway obstruction:
  - clear the airway
  - inflate the lungs
  - establish an alternative airway if needed.

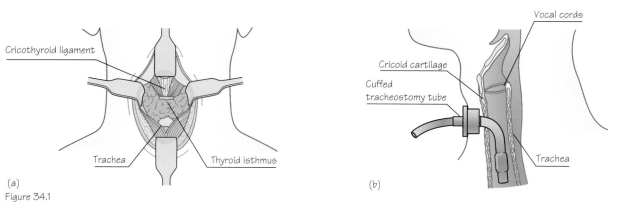

Cricothyroid ligament

Trachea

Thyroid isthmus

(a)

Vocal cords

Cricoid cartilage

Cuffed tracheostomy tube

Trachea

(b)

Figure 34.1

Performing a tracheostomy

The thyroid isthmus has been exposed ready to be divided (a). The next step would be to open the trachea between the second and fourth rings and insert the tracheostomy tube in the trachea below the vocal cords (b)

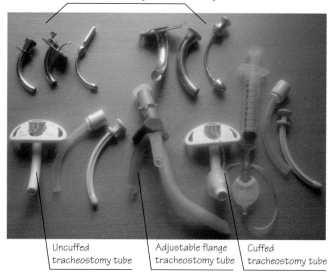

Paediatric and adult silver Negus tracheostomy tubes

Uncuffed tracheostomy tube

Adjustable flange tracheostomy tube

Cuffed tracheostomy tube

Figure 34.2

Tracheostomy tubes

Shown with their respective introducers and inner tubes

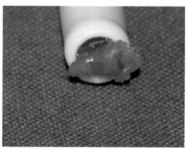

Figure 34.3

Tracheostomy tube lumen obstructed with a plug of dry secretions

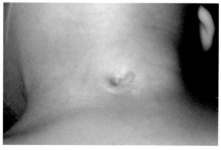

Figure 34.4

Child with a tracheo-cutaneous fistula after removal of a tracheostomy tube

Ear, Nose and Throat at a Glance, First Edition. Nazia Munir and Ray Clarke.

78 © 2013 Nazia Munir and Ray Clarke. Published 2013 by Blackwell Publishing Ltd.

Tracheostomy

Tracheostomy can be a life-saving operation and all doctors need to have knowledge of it.

Definitions

Tracheotomy is an opening in the trachea to permit air entry. A *tracheostomy* implies that the edges of the trachea have united with the skin of the neck to form a stoma or opening. Once the trachea has been opened it is usual to put a tracheostomy tube (Figure 34.1a,b) in the trachea to keep the hole open. This tracheostomy tube can then be attached to tubing for ventilation, used as a channel for suction catheters or attached to a speaking valve when the patient is well enough to be able to relearn speech (Figure 34.2).

Indications

There are many situations where a tracheostomy can be helpful, but most fall into one of the following categories:
1 Bypass airway obstruction
2 Permit respiratory toilet and suction
3 Help with artificial ventilation.
Some common causes of upper airway obstruction are shown in Figure 34.3.

Protecting the tracheobronchial tree and facilitating suction and ventilation can be especially important in very sick patients (e.g. following head trauma) or for patients who need to be managed on an intensive care unit with long-term artificial ventilation.

The procedure

Some of the principles of the procedure whereby a tracheostomy is fashioned are shown in Figure 34.1a,b. The operation is usually carried out under general anaesthesia with an endotracheal tube in place, but very rarely you may need to perform an emergency tracheotomy in an awake patient with local anaesthesia. This is a very fraught procedure, but can be life-saving.

The usual skin incision is made well above the sternal notch and the incision in the trachea (tracheotomy) is made between the second and fourth tracheal rings.

Types of tracheostomy tube

Figure 34.2 shows a range of tracheostomy tubes with their respective introducers and inner tubes. A cuffed tube is useful in the early stages following a tracheostomy (note the syringe for cuff inflation). The cuff can help protect the lower airway from secretions. In adults, an inner tube is easily removed for cleaning and to free the airway should the tube get blocked with secretions. In children, the tube may be too small to permit an inner tube. A 'speaking valve' diverts air into the larynx and pharynx during expiration and allows the patient to speak with the tracheostomy tube *in situ*. The silver tubes are now historical and used very infrequently as the newer plastic materials cause much less tissue irritation. The adjustable flange tubes are used in patients with an increased distance between skin and trachea because of body habitus or altered neck anatomy.

Aftercare

Tracheostomy patients need a lot of medical and nursing care especially in the early stages after the operation. They are often very ill, unable to cough and need frequent suction. As the air is taken straight into the trachea and bypasses the nose and mouth, it tends to be dry and needs to be humidified. This can be done by a humidifier attached to the tracheostomy tube or, in the later stages, use of saline sprays and nebulisers can be very helpful. Failure to ensure adequate humidification can cause thick secretions to dry out and form a cast that blocks the tube (Figure 34.3). It is important not to dislodge the tube for the first few days after the operation. By then the stoma or tract will have formed and it is much easier to change the tube.

Complications

Early complications occur at the time of surgery or shortly afterwards. Early complications of tracheostomy include the following:
• Bleeding: can be torrential if a large vessel in the neck is torn or erodes
• Pneumothorax (pleura is injured)
• Blockage of tube
• Dislodged tube.
Long-term complications include the following:
• Stenosis of the trachea, which can be especially problematic in children
• Voice and swallowing problems
• Persistent fistula, especially in children (Figure 34.4).

Clinical practice point

Do not wait until the patient is in extremis to perform a tracheostomy. If the patient has airway obstruction think of endotracheal intubation at an early stage and if this is likely to be prolonged consider a tracheostomy.

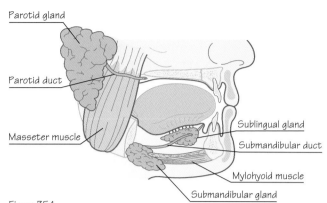

Parotid gland

Parotid duct

Masseter muscle

Sublingual gland

Submandibular duct

Mylohyoid muscle

Submandibular gland

Figure 35.1
The position of the main salivary glands

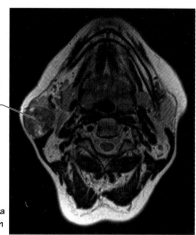

Right parotid lesion

Figure 35.2a
Axial MRI showing a right parotid lesion

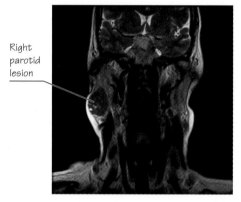

Right parotid lesion

Figure 35.2b
Coronal MRI showing a right parotid lesion

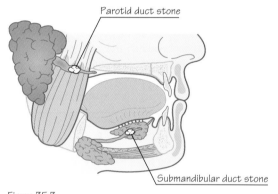

Parotid duct stone

Submandibular duct stone

Figure 35.3
Stones in the submandibular and parotid ducts

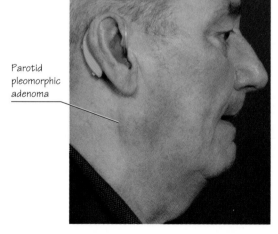

Parotid pleomorphic adenoma

Figure 35.4a
Lateral view of a right parotid pleomorphic adenoma

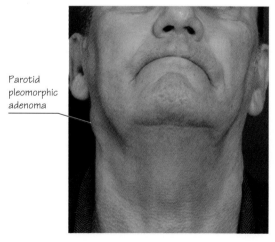

Parotid pleomorphic adenoma

Figure 35.4b
Antero-posterior view of a right parotid pleomorphic adenoma

Applied basic science

Saliva has an important role in starting the digestive process. It is also involved in maintaining good dental and periodontal health. It is produced by a series of glands in the mouth and pharynx. The major salivary glands are the parotid, submandibular and sublingual glands (Figure 35.1). The facial nerve runs through the parotid gland and is at risk in parotid surgery. Minor salivary glands are scattered throughout the mouth, tongue and soft and hard palates. Salivary enzymes, mainly amylase, are produced. The parotid gland produces saliva which leaves the gland by the parotid duct (also known as Stensen's duct) to enter the mouth opposite the second molar tooth. The duct forms a small papilla in the buccal mucosa through which saliva can be seen to pass when the mouth is inspected while massaging the gland. The submandibular gland secretes saliva through the submandibular duct (Wharton's duct) under the tongue on either side of the sublingual frenulum (see Figure 26.1b). The sublingual ducts secrete saliva through smaller individual ducts in the floor of the mouth (up to 20) and via the Wharton's ducts.

Examination and investigations

For examination of the neck see Chapter 28. Salivary gland pathology will often present with enlargement of one or more glands. The differential diagnosis includes other causes of neck swellings such as enlarged lymph nodes. When testing for enlargement of the submandibular gland it is useful to put your finger in the patient's mouth and see if you can feel the enlarged submandibular gland against another finger placed just under the mandible (bimanual palpation). Submandibular stones can also be felt in this way. Bimanual palpation can also be used to palpate the parotid papilla and duct for stones and masses in the anterior part of the parotid gland. No examination of the parotid glands is complete without evaluation of the facial nerve function by examining the muscles of facial expression.

Improved techniques in imaging in recent years have made the diagnosis of salivary gland pathology much more precise. Ultrasound examination, computed tomography (CT) and magnetic resoance imaging (MRI) scanning will give high-definition views of the major and minor salivary glands (Figure 35.2). Fine needle aspiration (FNA) biopsy in combination with radiological imaging can be very helpful in the investigation of parotid and submandibular lumps (see Chapter 29).

Salivary gland conditions
Inflammation of the salivary glands (sialadenitis)

Acute infection can cause swelling and abscess formation in the parotid or the submandibular glands. Most sialadenitis is obstructive in nature but the mumps virus causes swelling, particularly of the parotid glands. It is now much less common thanks to widespread vaccination but is increasing in recent years as a result of reduced uptake of the MMR vaccine because of concerns of autism related to the vaccine. Treatment of viral sialadenitis is symptomatic using analgesia, anti-inflammatory drugs and adequate hydration. Bacterial sialadenitis is seen in the elderly, usually when there is a degree of dehydration and poor oral care and hygiene. This is manifest by a diffuse, unilateral, acute onset, swollen parotid gland. The patient may be pyrexial. Examination reveals a tender, swollen and sometimes cellulitic parotid gland. Palpation will be very tender and inspection of the mouth during palpation often reveals thick mucopurulent secretions from the parotid duct. Treatment centres on scrupulous oral care and oral and systemic rehydration. Antibiotics have a role if cellulitis or abscess are suspected.

Salivary duct stones

Particles can precipitate in the salivary glands to form a stone (Figure 35.3). These are more prevalent in the submandibular duct but can also occur in the parotid duct. Patients present with recurrent swelling of the affected gland on eating or drinking, especially tart or sour food stuffs. The acute episode is treated with analgesics, locally applied heat and massage to reduce the swelling of the gland, but recurrent cases may require surgical removal of the stone. Stones can pass spontaneously into the mouth, but occasionally can reach sizes of up to 2 cm necessitating removal of the gland as well as the stone.

Salivary retention cyst

This is also referred to as ranula. The sublingual glands in the floor of the mouth can become swollen and cystic as a result of obstruction of the small ducts that empty into the mouth. This causes a retention cyst or ranula. Patients experience a persistent swelling under the tongue and, in large cases, under the chin in the submental area. A ranula is best treated by surgical removal.

Salivary gland neoplasm

The parotid gland is most often involved. The most common tumour is a benign pleomorphic adenoma (Figure 35.4a,b). Neoplastic lesions of the submandibular, sublingual and minor salivary glands are more likely to be malignant than parotid lesions. A high index of suspicion should be maintained to prevent misdiagnosis leading to delayed treatment. All discrete salivary masses should be thoroughly managed by a full history and examination, ultrasound-guided FNA and, in some cases, further imaging with MRI or CT scanning. Most salivary neoplasms, both benign and malignant, are treated surgically, with radiotherapy postoperatively in certain malignant tumours.

Dry mouth

A dry mouth is a common complaint in patients and can be brought about by a number of causes, including drugs, previous head and neck treatment (radiotherapy) and just not drinking enough fluid. This problem can be severe and can be associated with reduction in tear production by the lacrimal glands. This is known as sicca or Sjögren's syndrome and can be associated with inflammatory diseases such as rheumatoid arthritis or systemic lupus erythematosus. The aetiology is unknown and treatment can be very difficult. Artificial saliva and frequent fluids help to relieve dryness of the mouth; good dental care is essential to avoid dental caries.

Clinical practice point

Neoplastic lesions of the submandibular, sublingual and minor salivary glands are more likely to be malignant than parotid lesions. A high index of suspicion should be maintained.

---

36 The thyroid gland

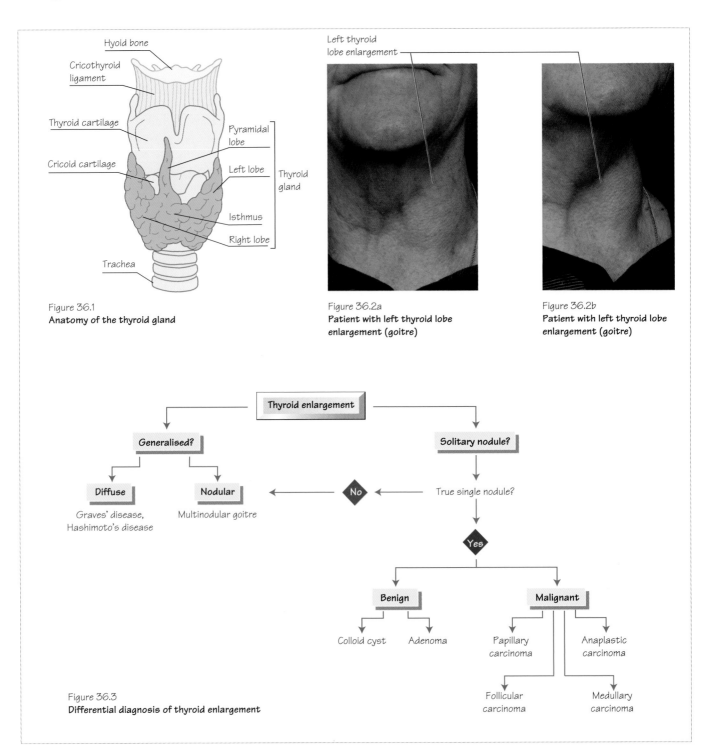

Figure 36.1
Anatomy of the thyroid gland

Figure 36.2a
Patient with left thyroid lobe enlargement (goitre)

Figure 36.2b
Patient with left thyroid lobe enlargement (goitre)

Figure 36.3
Differential diagnosis of thyroid enlargement

Anatomy

The thyroid gland is in the midline of the neck and is made up of the isthmus and two lobes (Figure 36.1). Some patients may also have a pyramidal lobe which is a normal developmental variant resulting from an embryological derivative of the thyroid gland. In the fetus, the gland is formed at the junction of the anterior two-thirds and posterior third of the tongue.

During intrauterine development, it descends down through the neck (through the region of the hyoid bone) to lie in its anatomical position. It takes with it a tract which obliterates in most people; if this does not close completely, a thryoglossal duct cyst may develop (see Chapter 29). Closely applied to the thyroid gland are the four parathyroid glands which produce parathyroid hormone. This is essential for calcium homeostasis.

Ear, Nose and Throat at a Glance, First Edition. Nazia Munir and Ray Clarke.

The gland is underneath the strap muscles of the anterior neck; these muscles help to move the larynx on swallowing. It overlies the trachea centrally, with the lobes of the gland wrapping round the sides to lie over the larynx and cricoid cartilages and the oesophagus and pharynx. The groove that lies between the trachea and the oesophagus is an important landmark as this is the location of the recurrent laryngeal nerve (see Chapter 31). The nerve is susceptible to damage in this region during thyroid surgery, which may result in a weak or breathy voice. A normal-sized thyroid gland is not usually visible but may be palpable; therefore, unless the thyroid is enlarged (a goitre) you will not see it externally in the neck (Figure 36.2).

Physiology

The thyroid gland is stimulated by thyroid stimulating hormone (TSH) from the pituitary gland to produce the thyroid hormones thyroxine (T4) and tri-iodothyronine (T3) by metabolism of dietary iodine. TSH has a negative feedback relationship with T3 and T4 – as the levels of T3 and T4 rise, secretion of TSH by the pituitary is inhibited and vice versa. The thyroid hormones are important in regulating growth and development both *in utero* and during childhood growth. In adults they regulate metabolism and have an important function in many of the body's physiological systems. Over-production of thyroid hormone is known as hyperthyroidism or thyrotoxicosis, and under-production of thyroid hormone is known as hypothyroidism. Thyroid function is assessed by performing blood tests. TSH assay alone can be informative of the patient's thyroid status because of the relationship between TSH and the thyroid hormones: if this is normal then the T3 and T4 levels are likely to be normal (euthyroid); if TSH is high then the T3 and T4 levels are likely to be low (hypothyroid); if the TSH is low then the T3 and T4 levels are likely to be raised (hyperthyroid). T3 and T4 blood levels can also be checked.

Presentation of thyroid pathology

Patients may present with signs and symptoms of hyperthyroidism or hypothyroidism, diffuse enlargement of the thyroid gland or lumps within the gland. Thyrotoxicosis causes sweating, hyperactivity, palpitations and poor sleep. Patients may have a tremor and tachycardia and complain of weight loss despite a normal or healthy appetite. This is often seen in auto-immune thyroid disease such as Graves' disease. This condition is often associated with thyroid eye disease manifest by exophthalmos, limitation of eye movements and lid lag. Hypothyroidism causes excessive sensitivity to cold, sleepiness, mental slowness, bradycardia and weight gain despite a poor appetite. Patients may develop alopecia and myxoedema. Hypothyroidism can occur as a normal physiological phenomenon with age, or after surgical removal of part or all of the thyroid gland.

Enlargement of the thyroid gland is termed a goitre but the term 'goitre' does not identify the actual cause of the enlargement (Figure 36.3). The enlargement may be caused by a smooth diffuse or a nodular increase in the size of the gland; both can occur with or without disorders of thyroid function. Generalised enlargement occurs in inflammatory conditions (thyroiditis) such as Graves' and Hashimoto's diseases. Nodular enlargement is a physiological change characterised by the development of multiple nodules of varying size over the whole of the gland – known as a multinodular goitre.

A solitary thyroid lump needs to be assessed to ascertain if it is truly a solitary lump or simply a dominant nodule within a multinodular goitre. Solitary nodules need to be investigated to exclude a thyroid malignancy; however, they may represent a simple cyst within the gland containing fluid (a colloid cyst) or a benign adenoma.

There are three main types of thyroid malignancy:
1 Papillary carcinoma
2 Follicular carcinoma
3 Anaplastic carcinoma.

Each affects patients in differing age groups: papillary carcinoma is predominantly seen in patients in their second to third decades, follicular cancer in patients over the age of 40 and anaplastic cancer in the elderly. Risk factors for thyroid cancer development include female sex, radiation exposure and a family history. Medullary carcinoma of the thyroid is often included as a thyroid cancer – this arises within the thyroid gland – but is a tumour of calcitonin-secreting C-cells rather than thyroid glandular tissue.

Investigation of thyroid lumps (see Chapter 29)

- Measure TSH ± T3 and T4 levels
- Thyroid auto-antibodies
- Ultrasound scan
- Fine needle aspiration (FNA) cytology with ultrasound guidance

Treatment

Hyperthyroidism may respond to anti-thyroid drugs (e.g. carbimazole) or can be treated with radioactive iodine. This treatment relies on the selective uptake of iodine by the thyroid gland to slow thyroxine production. Surgery may be required, but the patient then needs thyroxine replacement therapy indefinitely. Hypothyroidism needs to be treated with thyroxine replacement therapy. Multinodular goitres may require surgical removal if they are causing local compressive or cosmetic symptoms. Thyroid cancers are treated with surgical resection and postoperative radioactive iodine.

Clinical practice points

- The enlargement of all or part of the thyroid gland is the most common cause of a neck lump in adults.
- Investigation should be with blood tests, ultrasound ± fine needle aspiration cytology.

MCQs

1 The external ear
   a) is lined with ciliated columnar epithelium
   b) produces sweat
   c) may develop bony protruberances (exostoses) in response to extremes of temperature
   d) disorders can cause severe symptoms of imbalance
   e) is closed at birth

2 Otitis media
   a) is rare before the age of 1 year
   b) is often associated with complications
   c) is typically caused by anaerobic organisms
   d) infection can spread to the meninges
   e) in children, should prompt investigations to exclude HIV

3 Perforated eardrum
   a) causes severe deafness
   b) requires immediate repair to prevent intracranial sepsis
   c) often heals spontaneously
   d) cannot be caused by head trauma
   e) is often associated with facial palsy

4 Congenital deafness in children
   a) is best detected between the ages of 1 and 4 years
   b) can be caused by measles during the mother's pregnancy
   c) is more common in the industrialised world
   d) is usually reversible
   e) is more common in prematurity

5 Hearing aids
   a) work by stimulating the cochlea
   b) may cause distortion of sound
   c) are not suitable for very young children
   d) cannot be worn on both ears
   e) never cause wax to build up in the ear canal

6 Balance disorders
   a) are more common in the elderly
   b) steroids often produce dramatic improvement
   c) cannot be caused by diabetes mellitus
   d) if caused by inner ear disease, are never associated with tinnitus
   e) often need surgical treatment

7 Tinnitus
   a) is generally an ominous symptom of serious disease
   b) is more common in young adults
   c) responds well to treatment with sedatives
   d) needs urgent referral to an ENT department
   e) can be caused by aspirin

8 Facial palsy
   a) Bell's palsy is caused by a bacterial infection of the facial nerve
   b) steroids are contraindicated because of the risk of meningitis
   c) is usually painful
   d) may be complicated by keratitis
   e) cannot cause taste disturbance

9 Haematoma of the pinna
   a) is caused by a bleed in the ear canal
   b) pain is caused by pressure on the facial nerve
   c) is more common in males
   d) long-term deformity can be prevented by antibiotics
   e) is frequently idiopathic

10 Acute mastoiditis
   a) is more common in the elderly
   b) causes swelling of the pinna
   c) usually causes permanent hearing impairment
   d) may spread to the venous system and give rise to septic emboli
   e) surgery usually results in facial palsy

11 Adenoids
   a) are of maximum size in adolescence
   b) can be implicated in otitis externa
   c) cannot cause airway obstruction
   d) contain endocrine tissue
   e) may contribute to palatal closure

12 Acute sinusitis
   a) never involves more than one sinus (pansinusitis)
   b) complications include meningitis
   c) main organism is *Staphylococcus aureus*
   d) treatment is with anti-histamines
   e) is rare in the maxillary sinus

13 Deviated nasal septum
   a) is best corrected in early childhood
   b) is never caused by nasal trauma
   c) causes severe headaches
   d) can be caused by sinus infection
   e) surgery may cause long-term deformity

14 Nosebleeds
   a) may be fatal
   b) are more common in patients on anti-depressants
   c) do not respond to nasal cautery
   d) require nasal packing in most cases
   e) early surgery is the best approach in elderly patients

15 Allergic rhinitis
   a) is rare under the age of 5 years
   b) is associated with bronchial asthma
   c) is best managed with long-term oral steroids
   d) is caused by an excess of mast cells
   e) is more common in individuals with cystic fibrosis

16 Nasal fractures
   a) are more common in girls
   b) need immediate reduction for a good cosmetic result
   c) are not associated with mid-facial fractures
   d) may be complicated by a haematoma of the septum
   e) X-rays are essential to make the diagnosis

Ear, Nose and Throat at a Glance, First Edition. Nazia Munir and Ray Clarke.

17 Acute tonsillitis
  a) is more common in middle age
  b) does not affect swallowing
  c) cannot obstruct the airway
  d) requires hospital admission
  e) may cause mediastinitis

18 Tonsillectomy
  a) is mainly indicated to diagnose tonsillar cancer
  b) is not an accepted treatment for obstructive sleep apnoea
  c) is usually carried out under local anaesthesia
  d) may be indicated in children with two attacks of tonsillitis per year
  e) is no longer recommended for otitis media

19 The larynx
  a) is composed of bones and membranes
  b) closes and elevates during swallowing
  c) is innervated by the facial nerve
  d) is lined with ciliated epithelium throughout
  e) is behind the oesophagus

20 Laryngeal cancer
  a) is more common in men
  b) is associated with tobacco but not alcohol
  c) usually presents with airway obstruction
  d) is usually fatal
  e) spreads early to the liver

21 Hoarseness
  a) can be caused by accessory nerve injury
  b) may be caused by vocal cord nodules
  c) cannot be improved by speech and language therapy
  d) is an early sign of subglottic cancer
  e) may be a complication of parotid surgery

22 Enlarged neck nodes
  a) need urgent investigation in children
  b) are most commonly caused by tuberculosis
  c) can be a manifestation of HIV infection
  d) in laryngeal cancer, usually mean the tumour is inoperable
  e) are best investigated by CT scanning

23 The thyroid gland
  a) develops low in the mediastinum and migrates upwards
  b) produces parathyroid hormones
  c) is enlarged in iodine toxicity
  d) may be absent at birth
  e) reduces in size at puberty

24 Parotitis
  a) can be caused by mumps
  b) usually causes a painless swelling in the neck
  c) is less common in malnourished patients
  d) responds rapidly to treatment with aciclovir
  e) will usually require surgery to reduce complications

25 Tracheostomy
  a) is usually carried out as an emergency procedure under local anaesthesia
  b) involves making an incision in the laryngeal cartilages
  c) confines the patient to long-term hospital care
  d) can be complicated by a blocked tracheostomy tube
  e) is permanent if performed in children

26 Airway obstruction in children
  a) is characterised by a reduced respiratory rate
  b) steroids are an essential part of the management
  c) if caused by suspected epiglottiits, thorough examination of the throat is essential
  d) foreign body inhalation occurs mainly in adolescents
  e) may require an emergency operation to open the thyro-hyoid membrane

27 Neck abscess
  a) is most often caused by *Staphylococcus*
  b) is more common in elderly patients
  c) always needs surgery to drain pus
  d) complications include airway obstruction
  e) cannot spread to the mediastinum

EMQs

1 For the following diagram, identify the structures labelled from the options below. Each option can be used once, more than once or not at all.

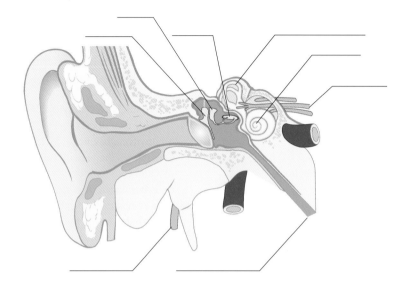

(a) Auditory nerve
(b) Cochlea
(c) Eustachian tube
(d) Facial nerve

(e) Incus
(f) Malleus
(g) Semicircular canal
(h) Stapes

2 For the following diagram, identify the structures labelled from the options below. Each option can be used once, more than once or not at all.

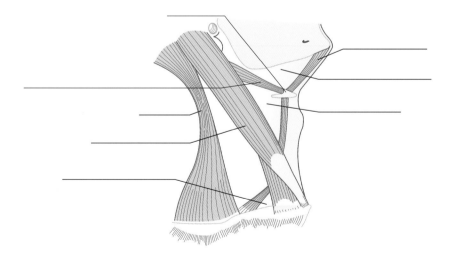

(a) Sternocleidomastoid
(b) Carotid triangle
(c) Submandibular triangle
(d) Hyoid bone

(e) Supraclavicular triangle
(f) Trapezius
(g) Anterior belly digastric muscle
(h) Posterior belly digastric muscle

Ear, Nose and Throat at a Glance, First Edition. Nazia Munir and Ray Clarke.

3 For the following diagram, identify the structures labelled from the options below. Each option can be used once, more than once or not at all.

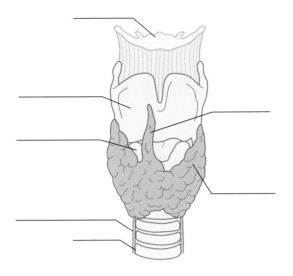

(a) Left thyroid lobe
(b) Recurrent laryngeal nerve
(c) Cricoid cartilage
(d) Pyramidal lobe of thyroid gland
(e) Trachea
(f) Hyoid bone
(g) Thyroid cartilage

4 For the following diagram, identify the structures labelled from the options below. Each option can be used once, more than once or not at all.

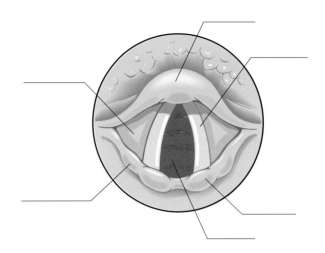

(a) Trachea
(b) Vocal cord
(c) Aryepiglottic fold
(d) Ventricular fold
(e) Epiglottis
(f) Arytenoid cartilage

5 For the following diagram, identify the structures labelled from the options below. Each option can be used once, more than once or not at all.

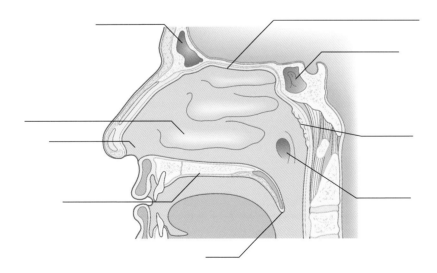

(a) Eustachian tube opening
(b) Inferior turbinate
(c) Sphenoid sinus
(d) Frontal sinus
(e) Hard palate

(f) Vestibule
(g) Cribriform plate
(h) Adenoids
(i) Uvula

Answers to MCQs

1 c
  a) The external ear is lined with keratinising stratified squamous epithelium
  b) It produces cerumen ('earwax')
  c) Correct. This is often seen in swimmers
  d) Imbalance is a result of inner ear disorders
  e) The external ear is fully open at birth. If not, this is microtia

2 d
  a) No, most common in this age group
  b) No, complications are serious but rare
  c) No, mainly pyogenic organisms (e.g. *Pneumococcus, Streptococcus pyogenes, Haemophilus*)
  d) Yes, meningitis can ensue. It is important to be alert to this
  e) No, otitis media is very common and investigation is only needed if the presentation is unusual or there are other features

3 c
  a) No, hearing is usually only slightly affected
  b) No, often heals itself and surgery is best deferred
  c) Yes, most perforations heal
  d) No, they can result from direct or indirect trauma
  e) No, this is very unusual

4 e
  a) No, early detection is vital, ideally at birth
  b) No, may be caused by German measles or rubella in the mother. Measles in the child can cause deafness
  c) No, more common in the developing world
  d) No, rarely from reversible causes
  e) Yes, prematurity is a risk factor

5 b
  a) No, they work by amplifying sound. Cochlear implants stimulate the cochlea
  b) Yes, can be a problem for hearing aid users
  c) No, used by babies as young as 2 weeks
  d) No, they can be worn in one or both ears
  e) No, they can cause wax build up. Many users complain of this

6 a
  a) Yes, much more common
  b) No, no real role for steroids
  c) No, imbalance can occur because of peripheral neuropathy, hypoglycaemia or hyperglycaemia
  d) No, tinnitus is often present (e.g. in Ménière's disease)
  e) No, very rarely needed

7 e
  a) No, mostly benign or idiopathic
  b) No, more common as people get older
  c) No, rarely appropriate
  d) No, unless there are unusual features (e.g. unilateral, other symptoms)
  e) Yes, this is a well-known side effect

8 d
  a) No, Bell's palsy is idiopathic
  b) No, they should be used in the early stages
  c) No, pain is rare, may suggest herpes zoster (Ramsay Hunt's syndrome)
  d) Yes, as eye closure can be affected
  e) Taste disturbance can occur because of involvement of the corda tympani nerve

9 c
  a) No, the bleed is between the layers of the pinna
  b) No, it is caused by pressure on the pinna itself
  c) Yes, because of their greater involvement in contact sports
  d) No, long-term deformity is brought about by necrosis of the cartilage and is best prevented by early aspiration
  e) No, caused by trauma (e.g. sports injury)

10 d
  a) No, mainly children
  b) No, the tissue behind the ear swells, the pinna is protruded forwards
  c) No, the prognosis for hearing is good
  d) Yes, this is a rare but serious complication
  e) No, the facial nerve is identified and preserved in mastoid surgery

11 e
  a) No, they increase in size up to the age of about 7 years
  b) No, otitis media
  c) No, they contribute to obstructive sleep apnoea
  d) No, lymphoid tissue
  e) Yes, especially in patients with cleft palate and can help with speech in this way

12 b
  a) No, often involves more than one sinus
  b) Yes, infection can spread intracranially
  c) No, mainly *Streptococcus pyogenes, Haemophilus influenzae, Streptococcus pneumoniae*
  d) No, anti-histamines are for allergic rhinitis
  e) No, this is the most common sinus involved

13 e
  a) No, surgery is best left until growth is complete
  b) No, a common cause
  c) No, very rare
  d) No, a deviated septum can *contribute* to sinus infection
  e) Yes, especially a saddle nose

14 a
  a) Yes, especially in older patients
  b) No, more common in patients on anti-coagulants
  c) No, nasal cautery is often effective
  d) No, most patients will not need a pack
  e) No, surgery is reserved for very troublesome, uncontrollable bleeding

15 b
  a) No, it is common in young children
  b) Yes, often the two co-exist
  c) No, very few people need long-term oral steroids. Topical steroids should be used first
  d) No, the mast cells degranulate but are not more numerous
  e) No, nasal polyps are more common but not allergic rhinitis

16 d
  a) No, more common in boys, who play more contact sports
  b) No, can be treated up to 2 weeks after the injury
  c) No, they are associated with mid-facial fractures
  d) Yes, important to look for this
  e) No, the important thing is to examine the nose carefully

17 e
  a) No, mainly children and young adults
  b) No, can make it painful to swallow
  c) No, airway obstruction is possible, especially in young children, and may need hospital admission and airway support
  d) No, most cases can be treated at home with analgesics and antibiotics
  e) Yes, rarely the infection can track through the neck tissues to the mediastinum

18 e
  a) No, the main indications are recurrent sore throat and obstructive sleep apnoea
  b) No, it is an acceptable treatment for obstructive sleep apnoea in children
  c) No, it is a painful operation and needs general anaesthesia
  d) No, guidelines recommend at least four to five attacks
  e) Yes, main indications now are sore throats and obstructive sleep apnoea

19 b
  a) No, it is composed of cartilages and membranes
  b) Yes, this is how aspiration of fluid into the lungs is prevented
  c) No, laryngeal nerves from the vagus
  d) No, the vocal cords are lined with squamous epithelium
  e) No, it is in front

20 a
  a) Yes, but women are catching up, probably because of smoking and alcohol use
  b) No, both are implicated
  c) No, this is unusual although it can occur
  d) No, the prognosis is good especially with early diagnosis
  e) No, liver metastases are late

21 b
  a) No, it can be caused by recurrent laryngeal or vagus nerve injury
  b) Yes, especially in singers
  c) No, speech and language therapy is an important part of management
  d) No, this cancer causes hoarseness late
  e) No, it can be a complication of thyroid surgery if the recurrent laryngeal nerve is damaged

22 c
  a) No, they are very common in children and only need investigation if unusual or persistent
  b) No, mainly viral infection
  c) Yes, persistent generalised lymphadenopathy can occur in patients with HIV
  d) No, surgery can be very effective even if the glands are involved
  e) No, CT is useful but ultrasound is easier and best as a first-line diagnostic tool

23 d
  a) No, it develops high and descends
  b) No, the parathyroid glands produce their own hormones
  c) No, iodine deficiency causes goitre
  d) Yes, the condition used to be called cretinism
  e) No, usually enlarges in puberty and in pregnancy

24 a
  a) Yes, mumps parotitis was well known before mumps vaccination
  b) No, parotitis is usually painful
  c) No, more common in malnourished patients because of dehydration and stasis of secretions
  d) No, rarely indicated
  e) No, treatment is usually medical

25 d
  a) No, mostly an elective procedure and under general anaesthetic
  b) No, the incision is well below the larynx
  c) No, many patients manage at home
  d) Yes, important to be aware of this
  e) No, usually reversible

26 b
  a) No, respiratory rate goes up
  b) Yes, dexamethasone is essential
  c) No, best not to examine the throat and cause spasm
  d) No, usually toddlers with a poor swallow and a tendency to put objects in the mouth
  e) No, *cricothyroid* membrane, as per APLS manual

27 d
  a) No, more likely *Streptococcus*, *Pnemococcus* or *Haemophilus*
  b) No, mostly children
  c) No, some can be managed with antibiotics
  d) Yes
  e) No, rarely can spread to mediastinum and can be fatal

Answers to EMQs

1

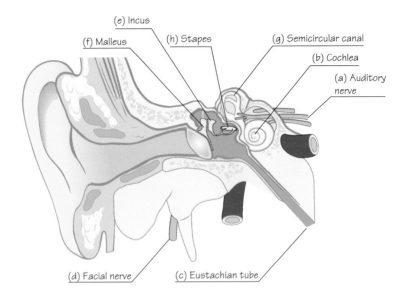

(e) Incus

(f) Malleus   (h) Stapes   (g) Semicircular canal

(b) Cochlea

(a) Auditory nerve

(d) Facial nerve   (c) Eustachian tube

2

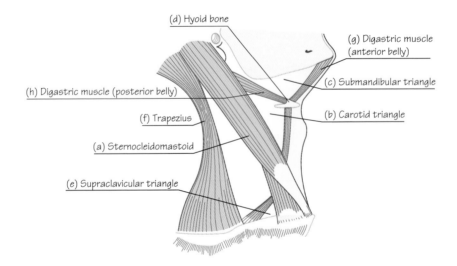

(d) Hyoid bone

(g) Digastric muscle (anterior belly)

(c) Submandibular triangle

(h) Digastric muscle (posterior belly)

(b) Carotid triangle

(f) Trapezius

(a) Sternocleidomastoid

(e) Supraclavicular triangle

3

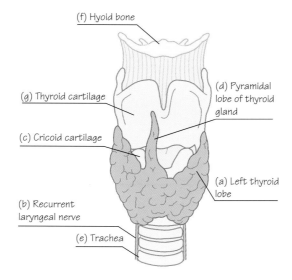

(f) Hyoid bone

(g) Thyroid cartilage

(d) Pyramidal lobe of thyroid gland

(c) Cricoid cartilage

(a) Left thyroid lobe

(b) Recurrent laryngeal nerve

(e) Trachea

4

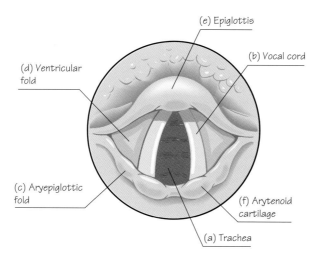

(e) Epiglottis

(b) Vocal cord

(d) Ventricular fold

(c) Aryepiglottic fold

(f) Arytenoid cartilage

(a) Trachea

5

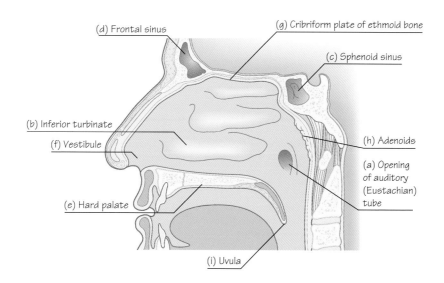

(d) Frontal sinus

(g) Cribriform plate of ethmoid bone

(c) Sphenoid sinus

(b) Inferior turbinate

(f) Vestibule

(h) Adenoids

(a) Opening of auditory (Eustachian) tube

(e) Hard palate

(i) Uvula

Index

Ear, Nose and Throat at a Glance, First Edition. Nazia Munir and Ray Clarke.